Color Atlas and Text of

DENTAL CARE
OF THE
ELDERLY

Color Atlas and Text of

DENTAL CARE OF THE ELDERLY

John R Drummond
BMSc, BDS, PhD
Lecturer in Dental Prosthetics and Gerontology

James P Newton
BSc, PhD, BDS
Senior Lecturer in Dental Prosthetics and Gerontology

Robert Yemm
BDS, BSc, PhD, FDSRCS(Ed.)
Professor of Dental Prosthetics Science

Department of Dental Prosthetics and Gerontology
The Dental School
University of Dundee
Scotland

M Mosby-Wolfe

London Baltimore Bogotá Boston Buenos Aires Caracas Carlsbad, CA Chicago Madrid Mexico City Milan Naples, FL New York Philadelphia St. Louis Sydney Tokyo Toronto Wiesbaden

Copyright © 1995 Times Mirror International Publishers Limited

Published in 1995 by Mosby-Wolfe, an imprint of Times Mirror International Publishers Limited

Printed by Grafos S. A. Arte sobre papel, Barcelona, Spain

ISBN 0 7234 1710 5

For full details of all Times Mirror International Publishers Limited titles, please write to Times Mirror International Publishers Limited, Lynton House, 7–12 Tavistock Square, London WC1H 9LB, England.

A CIP catalogue record for this book is available from the British Library.

Library of Congress Cataloging-in-Publication Data applied for.

Project Manager:	Mike Meakin
Developmental Editor:	Lucy Hamilton
Cover Design:	Pete Wilder
Production:	Mike Heath
Index:	Jill Halliday
Publisher:	Geoff Greenwood

Contents

CONTRIBUTORS

Dr B.J. Baum,
National Institutes of Health, Bethesda, U.S.A.
(Chapter 4)

Dr J.R. Drummond,
University of Dundee, Scotland.
(Chapters 1 and 4)

Dr A.S.T. Franks,
Central Birmingham Health Authority,
Birmingham, England.
(Chapter 15)

Professor P-O. Glantz,
University of Lund, Sweden.
(Chapter 8)

Professor A.R. Grieve,
University of Dundee, Scotland.
(Chapter 9)

Professor M.R.P. Hall,
University of Southampton, England.
(Chapter 2)

Dr M.J. Kowolik,
Indiana University, Indianapolis,USA.
(Chapter 6)

Professor P.J. Lamey,
Queen's University, Belfast, N. Ireland.
(Chapter 13).

Dr M.A.O. Lewis,
University of Wales, Cardiff, Wales.
(Chapter 13)

Mr I.J. McClure,
Perth Royal Infirmary, Perth, Scotland.
(Chapter 14)

Mr F.C. McManus,
University of Dundee, Scotland.
(Chapter 10)

Dr M.E.T. McMurdo,
University of Dundee, Scotland.
(Chapter 3)

Dr G.H. Moody,
University of Edinburgh, Scotland.
(Chapter 13)

Dr J.P. Newton,
University of Dundee, Scotland.
(Chapter 4)

Dr K. Nilner,
University of Lund, Sweden.
(Chapter 8)

Mr D.M. Quinn,
University of Dundee, Scotland.
(Chapter 10)

Dr G. Reddick,
University of Manchester, England.
(Chapter 5)

Dr E.M. Saunders,
University of Dundee, Scotland.
(Chapter 7)

Professor W.P. Saunders,
University of Glasgow, Scotland.
(Chapter 7)

Dr A. Schmitt,
University of Toronto, Canada.
(Chapter 12)

Professor R. Yemm,
University of Dundee, Scotland.
(Chapter 11)

Professor G.A. Zarb,
University of Toronto, Canada.
(Chapter 12)

PREFACE

The requirement, in many countries, for the dental profession to concentrate on treating the effects of dental caries in children is diminishing. This is fortunate, because of the concurrent though unrelated increase in both numbers and proportions of elderly people in the population. The similarity in timing of these two changes should allow resources to be transferred from care of young to care of old. However this is not a change which is easily achieved. In many respects, the older patient is not 'just an older adult', as a senior colleague remarked a few years ago.

The range of variation between individuals – never negligible, even in the very young – increases with age. Some of this variation is a consequence of the different effects of ageing itself, some a consequence of environmental and social factors, and some due to disease and illness experience (which can be environmentally influenced).

For dentistry, this requires careful assessment of each older person to help in the formulation of a strategy for care. It is often said that eating is a lasting pleasure in life. Whatever the truth of this, there is no doubt that maintenance of comfort, self respect and social freedom are all important goals to which the dental profession must contribute.

This text and atlas attempts to identify the population changes relating to elderly people, and to describe their characteristics. Successive chapters indicate how conventional views of 'adult' dentistry must be modified for management of the older person. In some aspects, and for some patients, it is necessary to revise downwards the objectives. For others, alternative techniques may provide scope for treatment results which are at least as successful as would be expected for younger patients.

A recurring theme in the chapters is the matter of maintenance. In many ways this is the key to successful continuing dental care of the elderly. In a high-caries society regular dental review was regarded as important for the young; the philosophy has a powerful attraction for the old. The fewer, and the smaller the risk of, unpleasant surprises and upsets of a stable equilibrium the better.

We hope that, in this book, we and our contributors have provided information on older people, on their varying needs and demands, and on the means of providing effective and sympathetic dental care. We hope also that the information will be of value to all sections of the dental profession. Adaptation of methods and skills to dentistry for the older age group is too important to be left to a section of the profession – it concerns all, from the youngest clinical student to the most senior practitioner.

ACKNOWLEDGEMENTS

We wish to acknowledge the efforts of all the contributors to this book, not only for the written word, but also for the excellent illustrations. We are sure that they, in turn, would wish us to record thanks for the efforts of photographers, radiographers and medical artists.

Our very great personal thanks are due to Miss M. O'Brien for her sterling work and patience during production of the manuscript, coping with revisions, rearrangements and a plethora of medical and technical terms

1. The Changing Populations of Elderly People

Interest in dentistry for the elderly and recognition that particular problems arise in treating the elderly has developed rapidly over the last few decades. Increasing numbers of undergraduate dental schools have well-developed geriatric dental courses and some have postgraduate programmes. The increasing time and other resources being devoted to treating elderly people is principally related to demographic changes in the population. An increasing proportion of the world's population is made up of elderly people, many of whom have considerable need for complex medical and dental care. In the more developed countries of the world there has been an increased retention of heavily restored natural teeth into old age. This has increased treatment needs considerably compared with the elderly person who is edentulous, where maintenance can be relatively straightforward. The increased retention of teeth in the elderly is partly as a result of better dental care and the increased use of preventive regimes. Another important factor in the elderly retaining, rather than losing, teeth in old age is the change in the elderly person's attitude to dental care. In many countries where previously elderly patients would have accepted readily the removal of natural teeth and the provision of dentures, this is no longer the case. Elderly patients today are much better informed of the various treatment options available to retain natural teeth and may also be more willing to devote their own resources to achieving this.

The elderly population of the United Kingdom has shown an increase in numbers from the beginning of the century and this trend is predicted to continue into the next century (**1**). It should be noted that the numbers of elderly in the United Kingdom will increase very little from now until the end of the century but will then continue to increase fairly sharply again. As in many countries the United Kingdom has seen an increase in the proportion of elderly in the population which has a significant effect on the social and economic organisation of the

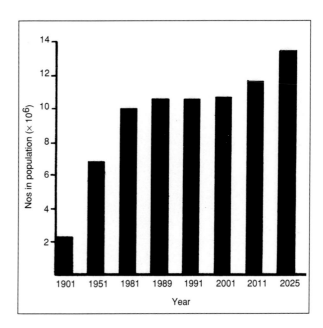

1 Population figures for the United Kingdom from 1901 predicted to 2025 (millions) – elderly people (males 65 years+, females 60 years+).

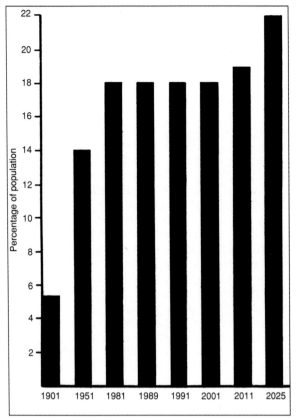

country. The changing proportions of elderly people in the United Kingdom are shown in **2,** and it should be noted that the proportion of elderly people will remain fairly static for the remainder of this century. However, a dramatic increase in the proportion of the elderly has occurred since about 1900. The proportion of elderly people in the population is predicted to increase significantly again in the next century. Another important change in the United Kingdom's population is the increasing numbers of those over the age of 75 years (**3**). The percentage of all elderly people who are over the age of 75 years has continued to increase steadily this century and is predicted to continue to increase well into the next century. The very elderly are a group who tend to make extremely heavy demands, in terms of medical and social provision. At present, in the United Kingdom at least, members of this very elderly group are mainly edentulous but increasing numbers will in the future retain natural teeth (see Chapter 5).

2 Elderly people (males 65+, females 60+) as percentage of population from 1901 to 2025 (predicted) for the United Kingdom.

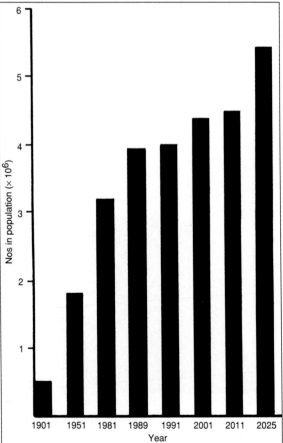

3 Numbers (millions) of very old (75 years+) in United Kingdom from 1901 and predicted to 2025.

In the United States there has also been an increase in the numbers (**4**) and proportion of elderly people. The increase has been dramatic, and it is striking to note that at the beginning of this century only around 3 million Americans were over the age of 65 years. By 2030 it is predicted that in the United States over 8.5 million people will be over 85 years of age.

In Europe there has also been an increase in the proportion of the population over the age of 65 years (**Table 1**). It is often assumed, mistakenly, that increased numbers of elderly is a phenomena restricted to the more developed parts of the world;

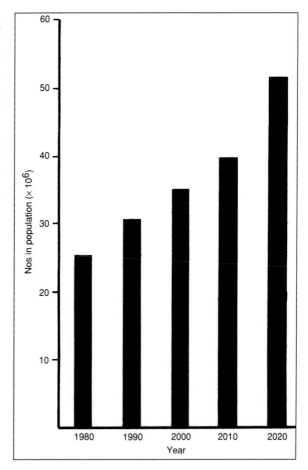

4 Numbers (millions) in the United States over age of 65 years from 1980 and predicted to 2020.

Table 1. Percentage of those in Europe over the age of 65 years from 1950 to 1990 with predictions for the next century to 2020.

Country	1950	1980	1990	2000	2010	2020
Austria	10.4	15.5	14.6	14.9	17.5	19.4
Belgium	11.0	14.4	14.2	14.7	15.9	17.7
Denmark	9.1	14.4	15.3	14.9	16.7	20.1
Finland	6.6	12.0	13.1	14.1	16.8	21.7
France	11.3	14.0	13.8	15.3	16.3	19.5
Germany	9.3	15.5	15.5	17.1	20.3	21.7
(Federal Republic as was)						
Greece	6.7	13.1	12.3	15.0	16.8	17.8
Iceland	7.6	9.9	10.3	10.9	11.2	14.2
Ireland	10.6	10.7	11.3	11.1	11.1	12.6
Italy	8.0	13.4	13.8	15.3	17.3	19.4
Luxemburg	9.8	13.5	14.6	16.7	18.1	20.1
Netherlands	7.7	11.5	12.7	13.5	15.1	18.9
Norway	9.5	14.8	16.2	15.2	15.1	18.2
Portugal	6.9	10.2	11.8	13.5	14.1	15.6
Spain	7.3	10.9	12.7	14.4	15.5	17.0
Sweden	10.2	16.3	17.7	16.6	17.5	20.8
Switzerland	9.6	13.8	14.8	16.7	20.5	24.4
Turkey	3.3	4.7	4.0	5.0	5.5	7.0
United Kingdom	10.7	14.9	15.1	14.5	14.6	16.3

Table 2. Numbers of elderly (millions) and percentage of population of elderly in developing countries in 1950 and 1980.

Region	1950		1980	
	Population	*Per cent*	*Population*	*Per cent*
Latin America				
60+ years	8.8	5.4	23.2	6.4
80+ years	0.6	0.4	2.2	0.6
Africa				
60+ years	12.1	5.5	22.9	4.9
80+ years	0.8	0.4	1.3	0.3
East Asia				
60+ years	50.6	7.5	103	8.7
80+ years	2.8	0.4	8.2	0.7
South Asia				
60+ years	54.1	7.6	71.1	5.1
80+ years	3.2	0.5	4.2	0.3

however, **Table 2** shows that in Africa, Latin America, East Asia and South Asia there has been a similar trend of increasing numbers of elderly people. There is a difference, however, in that in some countries the increasing elderly population has been more or less matched by an increase in other age bands (through high birth rate and lower infant mortality). Predictions (**Table 3**) suggest that proportions of elderly will increase in these regions in the future and that increases will be on a greater scale than those of the more developed countries.

The reasons for the increase in numbers and proportion of elderly are related to the increased life expectancy of the population and the low birth rate in certain parts of the world. It should be emphasised that the maximum lifespan of the human species has not changed significantly since records have been kept, but many more people now

Table 3. Predicted increase in numbers of elderly (millions) and percentage of population in 2000 and 2025.

Region	2000		2025	
	Population	*Per cent*	*Population*	*Per cent*
Latin America				
60+ years	41.0	7.3	93.3	10.8
80+ years	4.5	0.8	9.5	1.1
Africa				
60+ years	42.7	5.0	102	6.6
80+ years	2.8	0.3	8.2	0.5
East Asia				
60+ years	169	11.5	335	19.6
80+ years	17.0	1.2	31.1	1.8
South Asia				
60+ years	133	6.4	307	10.8
80+ years	8.0	0.4	22.1	0.8

survive into old age. One convincing example of increased longevity is the fact that in the United Kingdom in 1951 there were only around 200 centenarians, while today there are more than 4000. **Table 4** shows how life expectancy has increased in European countries while **Table 5** shows the increase in the United States. Even in the less developed countries life expectancy has increased dramatically this century. The other factor that has increased the proportion of elderly is the reduction in fertility levels, assessed by the average number of children per woman. This effect varies from country to country but in Europe declining fertility has certainly had a major effect on the age profile of the

Table 4. Changes in life expectancy in Europe from 1950–1955 to 1980–1985.

Country	Women		Men	
	1950–1955	*1980–1985*	*1950–1955*	*1980–1985*
Austria	68.4	76.7	63.2	69.5
Belgium	70.1	77.0	65.0	70.2
Denmark	72.4	77.6	69.6	71.5
Finland	69.6	78.0	63.2	69.8
France	69.5	78.7	63.7	70.6
Germany	68.3	76.8	64.4	69.7
(Federal Republic as was)				
Greece	67.5	76.0	64.3	72.1
Iceland	74.1	80.3	70.0	73.6
Ireland	68.2	75.7	65.7	70.4
Italy	67.8	78.0	64.3	71.2
Luxemburg	68.9	74.0	63.1	67.9
The Netherlands	73.4	79.5	70.9	72.7
Norway	74.5	79.5	70.9	72.6
Portugal	61.9	75.2	56.9	68.4
Spain	66.3	77.5	61.6	71.3
Sweden	73.3	79.4	70.4	73.4
Switzerland	71.6	79.7	67.0	72.8
Turkey	48.3	63.3	45.8	60.0
United Kingdom	71.8	76.9	66.7	70.7
Yugoslavia	59.3	73.5	56.9	68.0

Table 5. Life expectancy (years) at birth in United States of America 1920–1985.

Year	Males	Females
1920	53.4	54.6
1940	60.8	65.2
1960	66.6	73.1
1980	70.0	77.5
1985	71.2	78.8

Table 6. Average number of children per woman in 1900, 1965, 1975 and 1985.

Country	1900	1965	1975	1985
England and Wales	3.6	2.9	1.8	1.8
France	2.8	2.8	1.9	1.8
Finland	4.8	2.5	1.7	1.6
The Netherlands	4.5	3.0	1.7	1.5
Sweden	4.1	2.4	1.8	1.7
Switzerland	3.3	2.6	1.6	1.5

population. **Table 6** shows the decline in fertility levels in some European countries. In most of these countries fertility levels are now such that replacement of the generations is no longer possible, with an average of below two.

The changes in the age structure of the population will present a major challenge to the economic organisation of a nation's social services.

There is little doubt that medical and dental care of the elderly will continue to demand ever increasing resources and is likely to be more rather than less complex. With regard to dentistry there is little doubt that the attitude of the 'new' elderly is changing and the profession must be ready to meet this considerable challenge.

Further reading

Health Implications of Population Ageing in Europe. 1987. *World Health Statistics Quarterly*, **40**(1): 22–40.

Office of Population Censuses and Surveys (OPCS). 1989. *Population Projections 1989–2059 (1989 Based)*. HMSO, UK.

2. Characteristics of Older People

The normal elderly person?

This is really a philosophical question and therefore difficult to answer. What is elderly? The previous chapter has shown there to be an increase in the numbers of people who have reached retirement age. Some elderly, even the oldest, will be people who have normal physiological parameters, while others having many pathological changes and abnormal physiological responses will have variable degrees of disability. Are only those with normal physiology to be considered 'normal'? Obviously not, although they might be described as the physiological elite. Performance and functional ability are more important. Those who can lead independent lives of a quality that satisfies them are less likely to be a burden to their dependents and society. This has led to those older people being described as 'young old', while those who are dependent on help for their continuing survival are called the 'old old'. Alternatively the terms the Third Age or Fourth Age have been used, 'oldness' or 'age' being unrelated to chronological age. Old person's complaints are often attributed to their age; in other words thought by the health professional to be related to the ageing process. While this may be so, it can be used as an excuse for inaction. If the complaint usually indicates disability or discomfort in performing the activities involved with daily life: the individual has a problem. This may be resolved by alteration of life style, sophisticated medical or surgical treatment or a combination of solutions. Depending on the degree of disability or discomfort and the success of the remedy, the complainant may move from the Fourth Age to the Third Age or vice versa.

A 'normal' elderly person is one who can be categorised as belonging to the 'young old' or 'Third Age' group. This means that, regardless of their age or potential pathology, they are content with their functional ability and way of life. It does not mean that they have no remediable medical condition or that their lifestyle could not be improved by a variety of interventions. (5).

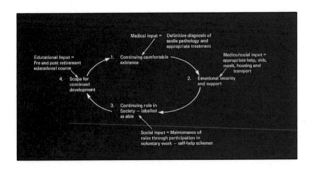

5 The positive life cycle – maintenance of good health in the elderly.

Ageing

The basic concept of ageing is loss of the organism's adaptability with time. However this is not an intrinsic property of all organisms which means that not all need to age (e.g. sea anenomes, microorganisms, plants, etc.). Biological research may uncover, in time, the intrinsic ageing processes. At present we do not know, although Pathy's textbook *Principles and Practice of Geriatric Medicine* devotes 162 pages to 'Scientific Aspects of Human Ageing'. Various mechanisms and theories of ageing have been proposed, suggesting the complexity of the problem and perhaps obscuring it (Comfort, 1979). Any theory must satisfy four criteria – the process must be intrinsic, deleterious, progressive and universal within the species. The most convincing theory to meet these criteria has been put forward by Kirkwood (1981). This is the disposable stroma theory which proposes that ageing results from the body's inability to repair random environmental damage. As a result, random defects occur in somatic cells and the additive effects of these results in senescence and death. Kirkwood (1988) maintains that this theory fits in with many postulated specific causes of damage as well as theories and mechanisms (**Tables 7, 8**). Ageing is therefore an intrinsic mechanism which is influenced by a whole series of extrinsic factors. The rate at which ageing occurs will therefore be slowed or accelerated by variation of these external events, although intrinsic genetic factors may also play a part, e.g. Werner's syndrome.

Studies of nonagenarians suggest that while genetic inheritance may play a part, social and other factors may be equally important. For instance, although there was a high incidence of longevity in the family history of nonagenarians studied, their place in the sibling order (either high or low) appeared to indicate that economic and nutritional factors may have also been influential. Recent studies involving dietary restriction in laboratory rats and mice have shown that lifespan can be increased by as much as one third and that animals remain fertile longer, even though their litters are smaller.

As far as humans are concerned there has been little increase in life span (**6**), although many more people are reaching the age of 100 years. This means that the survival curve has altered its shape (**7**) so that it is becoming 'squared off'. As can be seen, 75% survival has risen from between 20–30 years in 1901 to 60–70 years in 1975. The effect has been mainly a result of the great improvement that has taken place in perinatal and infant mortality rates, reduction in poverty, better housing and public health measures.

As would be expected, death rates per 1000 have decreased in all age groups. Studies of hospital discharges confirm the increasing morbidity that occurs with age (**8, 9**). Considerable evidence is accrueing from intervention studies that morbidity can be reduced and lifestyle improved (Rose, 1985). Compression of morbidity is occurring: a state in which the increase in the age-specific incidence of chronic disease markers is more rapid than the increase in life expectancy (Fries, 1983). In other words people are staying fitter for longer and the terminal phase of ageing (Svanborg *et al.*, 1988) is becoming shorter and more obvious.

Table 7. Mechanisms that may be affected by failure of maintenance.

1. Cell replacement and wound healing.
2. Repair of DNA damage.
3. Accuracy of DNA, RNA and protein synthesis.
4. Degradation of defective proteins.
5. Removal of free radicals.
6. Immune response to infections.
7. Detoxification.
8. Stability of differentiated or stem line cells.

Table 8. Theories of ageing.

1. Stomatic mutations.
2. Protein errors.
3. Denatured proteins.
4. Free radicals.
5. Immunological failure.
6. Epigenetic defect.
7. Toxic products.

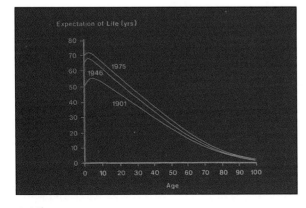

6 Life span.

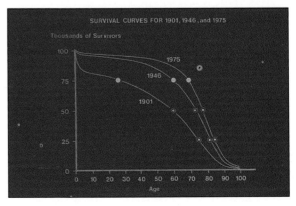

7 Survival curves.

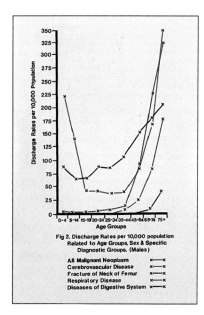

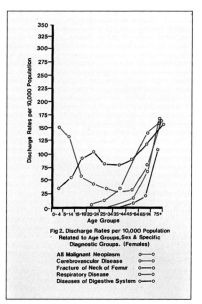

8 Hospital discharge rates (Males).   **9** Hospital discharge rates (Females).

Some physiological changes

The reduction that occurs in some physiological parameters is shown in **10**. However, it should be pointed out that the measurements recorded are average, point-in-time measurements taken from groups of age-related healthy volunteers. Consequently they represent age differences between groups. They are not necessarily age changes, for we do not know what the oldest age groups average measurements would have been at earlier intervals in their life. There can be considerable overlap between values found in the old with those found in the young. As can be seen in **11**, renal diodrast clearance diminishes with age but values for some of the 70-year-olds are as high as those for the young. Obviously, physiological changes in organs and systems will have various effects. Such deterioration in renal function could affect the excretion of toxic waste products as well as medicines and drugs, yet as **11** shows this does not apply to all elderly. Histological changes occur

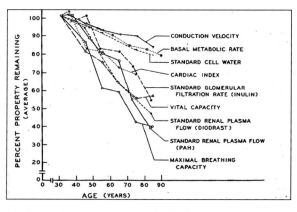

10 Reduction in some physiological parameters.

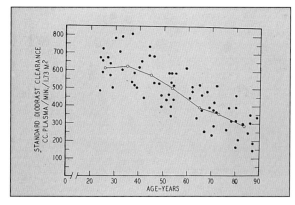

11 Reduction in standard renal diodrast clearance.

in the renal glomerulus, with the basement membrane becoming thickened (**12, 13**) and those undoubtedly contribute to any physiological deficit.

Cohort studies are beginning to establish reference values for various biochemical, psychological and physiological parameters and to demonstrate true age changes. These studies confirm that functional measures vary considerably in their response to time (age). Some functions begin to decline almost as soon as growth and development is complete, while others may be well-preserved at 70 years or older. This particularly applies to psychological functions, some, like psycho-motor speed, deteriorate early while intellectual parameters such as vocabulary may still

be improving in old age. An effect of such a deficit leads to slowness of response and may manifest itself as an inability to make up one's mind. Decline in some functions therefore follows a two-phase curve, while in others it presents a more complex pattern, which Svanborg (1988) suggests has four phases (**14**). Even then, caution is needed for the old adage 'if you don't use it you'll lose it' still holds. The Göteborg study has shown that if 75-year-old people train, the appearance of their striated muscle alters, its function increasing, thereby improving strength and stamina (Aniansson *et al.*, 1983). Similarly, others have shown that exercise capacity, as measured by maximum oxygen intake (V_{O_2} max), can be maintained by training and consequently

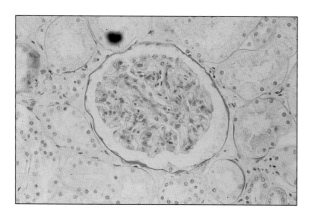

12 Histological appearance of renal glomerulus in 22-year-old (Periodic acid–Schiff's (PAS) stain).

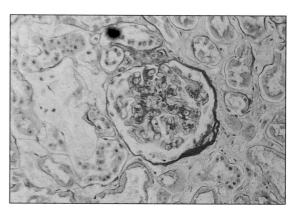

13 Histological appearance of renal glomerulus in 87-year-old (Periodic acid–Schiff's (PAS) stain).

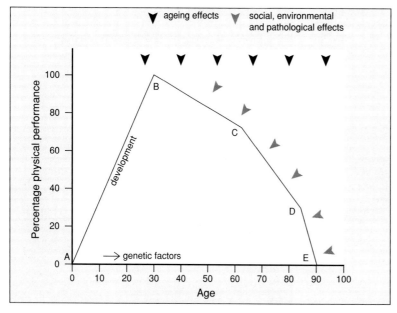

14 Drawing of four-phase pattern of life-long 'performance', assuming 100% performance at 30 years. Slopes of BC and CD will vary; DE will become more vertical.

stamina (**15**). Moreover, the inactive can achieve the levels of the active if they train; the worse one is the easier it is to improve. The effect of keeping in training undoubtedly maintains function and therefore quality of life, but may only prolong the third phase and shorten the fourth.

Exercise has a beneficial effect on many physiological parameters, particularly cardiorespiratory. Pulmonary function diminishes in old age as a result of disease, as well as alteration of elastic tissue (**16**). Similarly, mean blood pressure rises (**17**) owing to increasing inelasticity of the arterial wall. The fact that mean blood pressure appears to be lower in the very old is probably due to a cohort effect; those with lower blood pressures at younger ages survive longer.

Biochemical and physiological changes in the central nervous system (CNS) may give rise to changes in behavioural capacity. These may be exaggerated by disease, as well as social and environmental factors. As previously indicated old people are not as quick and deft as the young

although there will be considerable variation. 'Sway' is a good measure of coordination and balance, and it can be demonstrated that this diminishes during growth and development and then deteriorates with age (**18**). The reduction in the conduction velocity of nervous tissue (**10**) means that it is more difficult to correct errors in movement and the individual is unable to react when a faster response is needed. The risk of falling is increased and this, coupled with other factors such as diminution of the visual field, will increase environmental hazards, e.g. crossing the road.

The special senses of vision, hearing, taste and smell, all tend to be reduced in old age. Only part of this reduction can be attributed to the ageing process. Disease, social and environmental factors all play a part. It is obvious that loss of any or all of these, to a greater or lesser degree, will have an effect on the quality of an individual's life. This can lead to mental illness, e.g. depression, paraphrenia. Deafness is particularly common affecting about 30% of the over 65 years population. Being hard of

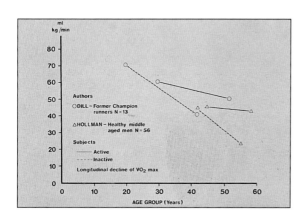

15 Loss of physical capacity.

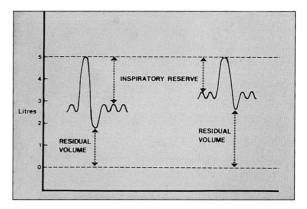

16 Spirogram to show loss of lung function (young on left, old on right).

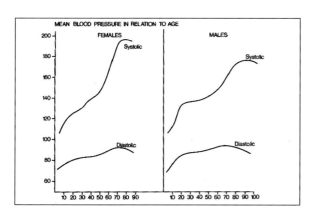

17 Diagram to show mean blood pressure in relation to age.

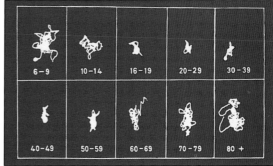

18 Effect of age on 'Sway'. Typical tracings from each age group in a direct vision/stance test (age in years).

19

hearing increases with age (**19**). It can lead to isolation because of the inability to communicate; this is a result of the loss of high frequency sound, so that only the lower frequency elements of speech (normal range 50–200 Hz) are heard, and decoding language becomes difficult. Correcting this deficit by amplification is only partly successful and overamplification (shouting) may actually be painful.

Alteration in the size of body compartments (**20**) has an affect on various biochemical and physiological values. In addition, changes in metabolism occur. Loss of tissue means that some body reserves are lost, although these reserves are usually so large that the losses rarely matter. For example, serum potassium levels remain the same in young and old despite reduction in total body potassium, reflecting loss of cellular tissue (**21**).

Control of body sugar is an example of how the body's ability to regularise homeostasis diminishes. The response to a glucose load alters with age (**22**), the peak occurring later in the 9th to 10th decade, at 1 hr. Similarly, the insulin response is later and the area under the curve in both instances increases. This translates into an inability to control blood sugar level when individuals are studied throughout the day. The blood sugar levels in the young stay almost constant with insulin peaks following the main meals, while the levels remain high in the old despite higher insulin responses (**23**). This may not matter, but the incidence of type II diabetes mellitus rises with age and occurs in subjects with normal fasting blood sugar levels (**24**).

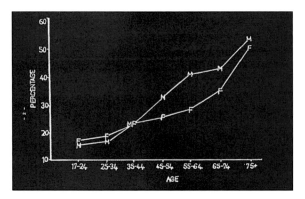

19 Difficulty in hearing with age: percentage of males (M) and females (F) reporting hearing difficulty in conversation.

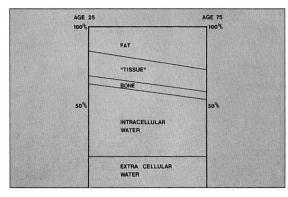

20 Alteration in the size of body compartments with age.

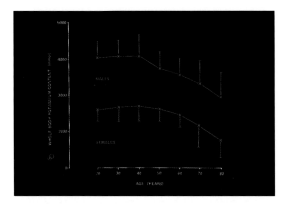

21 Reduction in whole body potassium content with age. (Courtesy of Professor M. D. W. Lye.)

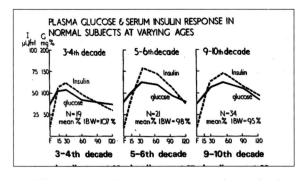

22 Effect of age on the response to 50 g glucose load.

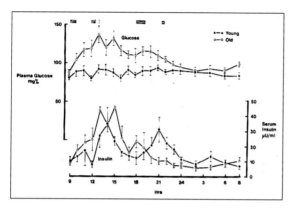

23 Effect of age on blood sugar control in normal subjects. (Courtesy of Professor G. Alberti.)

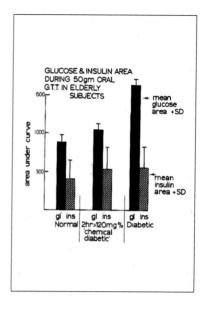

24 Response of 'normal' 85-year-old elderly subjects to 50 g oral glucose load.

Disease, environment, social factors and adaptation

The part that disease, the environment and social factors play in ageing has already been indicated (**5**). How the individual adapts biologically, socially and psychologically to those factors will be reflected in their oldness, which has no relation to their chronological age. The effect of disease on two 85-year-old identical twins is shown in **25**. Both suffer from diseases with an immunological background which has triggered a different response in each individual. The lady on the left has hypothyroidism with a high titre of anti-thyroid antibodies. While the lady on the right has rheumatoid arthritis with a high rheumatoid factor level. Her shrunken appearance is a result of the collapse of her thoracic vertebrae from associated osteoporosis, which has been induced by immobility and previous steroid therapy. As has previously been indicated, disuse is followed by atrophy. Exercise, as well as being beneficial with regard to activity and stamina, will help to prevent bone loss and development of osteoporosis. Diseases that affect mobility, such as the arthropathies, will therefore have other effects on the human organism; these may be direct effects on other physiological systems, or indirect in that they may require social and environmental adjustments. Adaptation to those direct or indirect effects will influence the ageing of that particular individual. Similarly, other factors may influence the occurrence of a disease process. It would seem probable that the greater the bone mass when young the lesser the risk of bone fracture when old. Matkovic *et al.*, (1979) report a comparison of two Yugoslavian districts. In one the calcium intake was high in the other low; the prevalence of hip fractures was lower in the district with the high intake.

Similarly, other social and environmental factors will have an effect on how an individual ages. There can be no doubt that poverty has a considerable effect, and the low life expectation in the third world is not only due to high perinatal and infant mortality, but also to poor national infrastructures, resulting from lack or misuse of gross national product. In other words, clean water, better hygiene and sanitation, good agricultural policies and an efficient health service will alter the ageing profile of the population. It has been suggested that the increase in life expectancy in Japan is a result of strong health service programmes, which, it is claimed, decrease the demand for inpatient care for the

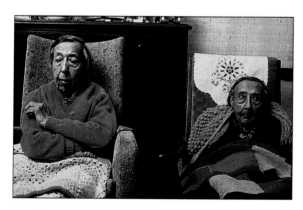

25 Identical twins aged 85 years.

elderly (Tatara *et al.*, 1991). These social and environmental factors need to be taken into account when analysing cohort studies. What has happened earlier in the life of individuals will have an effect on how they age. These can include war, economic depression, epidemic diseases, imprisonment, poor education, low occupational status or specific cultural demands with regard to life style.

Conclusion

The process of biological ageing has not yet been fully elucidated, but it seems probable that failure to repair somatic defects is a major cause. This process has been termed 'senescing'. It may be influenced by disease, the incidence of which increases as time progresses, and by the genetic make-up of the individual. Similarly, social factors will cause the person to adapt in a way acceptable to that society, i.e. 'eldering' or growing old socially. Finally, the individual will choose various types of behaviour in order to adapt to the environment, including the processes of senescing and eldering, thereby ageing psychologically (Woods and Birren, 1991). In this way, biological, social and psychological ageing will occur. While each territory is linked to the others, they do not necessarily bear any relation to chronological time. Hence, someone can be biologically young, socially middle-aged and psychologically young in advanced chronological age, e.g. over 90 years.

References

Aniansson, A., Sperling, I., Rundgren, A. & Lehnberg, E. 1983. Muscle function in 75-year-old men and women. A longitudinal study. *Scand. J. Rehabil. Med. Suppl.*, **9**, 92–102.

Comfort, A. 1979. *The Biology of Senescence* 3rd edn. Churchill Livingstone, Edinburgh.

Fries, J.F. 1983. The compression of morbidity. *Millbank Mem. Fund Q.*, **61**, 397–419.

Kirkwood, T.B.L. 1981. Repair and its evolution: survival versus reproduction. In *Physiological Ecology: An Evolutionary Approach to Resource Use*, eds C.R. Townsend & P. Carlow, pp. 165–89. Blackwell Scientific Publications, Oxford.

Kirkwood T.B.L. 1988. The nature and causes of ageing. In *Research and the Ageing Population. Ciba Foundation Symposium 134*, pp. 193–207. John Wiley and Sons, Chichester.

Matkovic, V., Kostial, K., Simonovic, I., Buzina, R., Brodarec, A. & Nordin, B.E.C. 1979. Bone status and fracture rates in two regions of Yugoslavia. *Am. J. Clin. Nutr.* **32**, 540–9.

Pathy, M.S.J. (ed.). 1991. *Principles and Practice of Geriatric Medicine*, 2nd edn. John Wiley and Sons, Chichester.

Rose, G. 1985. Role of controlled trials in evaluating preventive medicine procedures. In *The Value of Preventive Medicine. Ciba Foundation Symposium 110*, pp. 183–202. Pitman, London.

Svanborg, A. 1988. The health of the elderly population: results from longitudinal studies with age-cohort comparisons. In *Research and the Ageing Population. Ciba Foundation Symposium 134*. John Wiley and Sons, Chichester.

Svanborg, A., Berg, S., Mellström, D., Nilsson, L. & Persson, G. 1988. Possibilities of preserving physical and mental fitness and autonomy in old age. In *Mental Health in the Elderly. A Review of the Present State of Research*, ed. H. Hafner, pp. 195–202 Springfield, Berlin/Heidelberg.

Tatara, K., Shinsho, F., Suzuki, M., Takatorige, T., Nakanishi, N. & Kuroda, K. 1991. Relation between use of health check ups in middle age and demand for inpatient care by elderly people in Japan. *Brit. Med. J.* **302**, 615–18.

Woods, A.M. & Birren, J.E. 1991. The psychology of ageing. In *The principles and Practice of Geriatric Medicine*, 2nd edn, ed. M.S.J. Pathy. John Wiley and Sons, Chichester.

3. Medical Problems in the Elderly

General Considerations

Atypical presentation

The presentation of many disease processes in the elderly may be very different from that of younger counterparts and tends to be more muted or less acute. The perception of pain, for example, appears to be altered in some old people in certain disease states, hence the 'silent' or painless myocardial infarction, or the painless perforation of a duodenal ulcer.

Infections, such as pneumonia, may occur in the absence of a pyrexia or a leucocytosis, and present instead with immobility, falls or confusion. Indeed, given the impairment of postural reflexes present in many old people, almost any disease may present with falls or impaired mobility.

Multiple pathology

In contrast to younger patients, the simultaneous coexistence of several illnesses is the norm in old age. Some of the illnesses may be of a minor nature, but nonetheless impinge on the person's overall well-being. This phenomenon of multiple pathology occurs for several reasons (**Table 9**).

Table 9. Reasons for multiple pathology in the elderly.

1. Diseases with long latent periods	e.g. vascular diseases.
2. Age-related increase in incidence of certain diseases	eg. diabetes mellitus, cancer
3. Age-related decline in immune function	Autoimmune disorders, e.g. pernicious anaemia, thyroid disease
4. Complications of immobility	e.g. deep venous thrombosis, broncho-pneumonia, impaired homeostasis

Homeostasis

With ageing and cumulating pathologies, reserve capacity to protect performance and restore equilibrium is diminished. Ageing produces a decline in the ability to adapt to changes in the internal or external environment.

Infections

An increased morbidity and mortality owing to infection occurs in the elderly. This is believed to be due to a deterioration in the inflammatory and immune responses with ageing, and also to the occurrence with an age-related incidence which enhance susceptibility to infection. Bacterial infections particularly pneumonias, endocarditis and hospital-acquired infection are more likely to be lethal in this age group. In addition, certain specific infections appear to be more common in the elderly, for example tuberculosis and *Herpes zoster* (**26**). Both of these conditions may represent reactivation of a long-dormant infection, which re-emerges with the waning vigour of the ageing immune system.

Falls

Falls represent a major threat to the health and independence of the elderly population, and often signify the presence of a serious underlying disorder. The likelihood of falling increases with age, as does the risk of fracture and death. Normal balance depends on local reflexes and the central co-ordination of information from the lower limbs, proprioceptors, eyes and vestibular mechanisms.

Epidemiology

A major study showed that one-third of the population aged 65 years and over had sustained one or more falls within the preceding year. Surveys of old people living in institutions have reported an even higher incidence. Most falls do not result in serious physical injury, and only 6% of falls are thought to result in fracture. Women fall more than men. Other characteristics associated with a high likelihood of falling are living alone, the presence of chronic illness, impaired mobility, and postural instability.

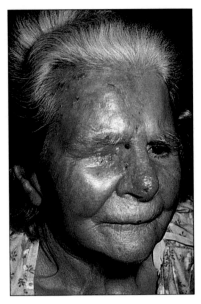

26 Ophthalmic *Herpes zoster* (shingles).

Complications

Falls may result in a variety of physical complications, including bruising and laceration, fracture, hypothermia, pressure sores, dehydration and bronchopneumonia.

It is important to emphasise, however, that even if a fall does not result in physical injury, the psychological implications may be devastating. The shock of falling, together with a fear of future falls, may lead to a debilitating loss of confidence and deliberate restriction of daily life, and renders many old people housebound.

Cause of falls

Environmental

Elderly people often live in old, poorly illuminated cramped accommodation. The clutter of rugs, electrical wiring, walking frames and pets conspire to produce accidents and falls in the home.

Drugs and alcohol

Many of the commonly prescribed hypnotics, tranquilliser and antidepressant drugs produce sedation and unsteadiness. Postural hypotension resulting from the prescription of a diuretic may be implicated as a cause of falls. Alcohol consumption can have similar effects.

Sensory impairment

The control of posture requires intact vestibular, visual and proprioceptive mechanisms, and the elderly brain is less efficient at integrating the various inputs and outputs required for perfect balance.

Locomotor

Disorders affecting the muscles and joints, for example osteoarthritis, and neurological conditions like Parkinson's disease and stroke, all increase the risk of falling.

Impaired cerebral perfusion

Intermittent disturbance of cardiac rhythm, a postural drop in blood pressure and transient strokes all temporarily impede cerebral blood supply, and may result in falls.

Vision

As age progresses, the cornea becomes gradually more opaque, the lens loses much of its accommodating power, and the most sensitive part of the retina, the macula, loses some of its colour perception abilities. Deposition of calcium and cholesterol salts at the limbus (arcus senilis) is a common finding in the elderly (**27**).

The majority of diseases leading to visual disability occur in the elderly, and this is reflected in the high prevalence rates for both blindness and partial sight in this group. Between the ages of 75–79 years, some 1% are registered blind; over the age of 85 years the figure is 85%. The common eye diseases of old age in order of frequency are cataract, macular degeneration and glaucoma (**28**). All these conditions are amenable to treatment, particularly cataract, as surgical lens extraction and implantation may be successfully performed on even the frailest old person.

As most eye disease in the elderly is progressive, a stage is usually reached when the limitations imposed by poor sight, in conjunction with other disabilities, threaten independence. Research has demonstrated high levels of unreported, but eminently treatable visual problems among the elderly.

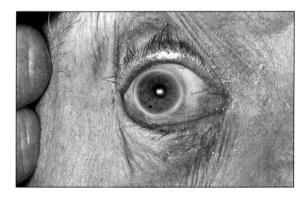

27 Arcus senilis.

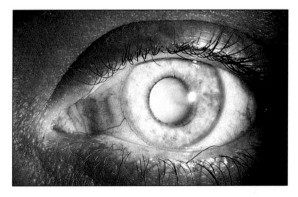

28 Cataract.

Hearing

Most elderly people suffer from a varying degree of hearing loss. Elderly males are affected more than females, and 60% of those aged 70 years suffer hearing impairment which makes communication difficult.

Speech consists of a wide range of sound frequencies (100–10000 Hz), the vowels being of low frequency while the consonants are weaker and of high frequency. In old age in general, higher frequencies are affected more than lower ones. The importance of this is that the high-frequency consonants are lost, whereas the lower-frequency vowels are retained, making speech difficult to understand. Shouting to deaf old people merely increases the volume of the low frequencies, which then become uncomfortable. This is exacerbated by loudness recruitment in which there is a disproportionate increase of loudness after a certain threshold of sound volume. This has a major disadvantage in that the unwanted loud sounds such as dogs barking and doors slamming are heard at the expense of wanted information such as speech.

The elderly are also less able to cope with fast speech than younger people.

Deafness is one of the least tolerated forms of impairment and causes a great deal of irritation and frustration, both for the patient and for those around him or her. Electronic hearing aids amplify sound and are sufficient to overcome the majority of communication barriers in elderly people.

Cardiovascular disease

Ischaemia is by far the commonest cause of heart disease in old age and ischaemic heart disease is a source of significant morbidity and mortality. Systemic hypertension (>160/>95 mmHg) is the most significant risk factor for the development of ischaemic heart disease in the elderly, and also predisposes them to stroke, peripheral arterial disease, hypertensive retinopathy and renal failure (**29**).

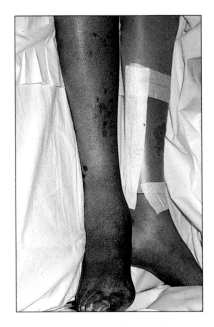

29 Peripheral arterial embolism.

Ischaemic heart disease

The disease is usually inferred from a history of angina or of myocardial infarction and is usually caused by atherosclerosis.

Men are affected more commonly than women, and the incidence rises with age. Cigarette smoking, hypertension, diabetes mellitus, obesity and hyperlipoproteinaemia are recognized risk factors.

Angina pectoris is a clinical diagnosis based on a typical history of central crushing chest pain, precipitated by effort (walking uphill), cold or emotion. The pain often radiates to the left arm and up into the jaw. Treatment is aimed at risk-factor modification and therapy with sublingual glyceryl trinitrate (GTN) tablets or spray. GTN is taken either to relieve pain, or prophylactically before known precipitating events. Anginal pain lasting more than 15 min, and resistance to two or three doses of GTN may represent a myocardial infarction and the patient should be referred immediately to hospital.

Myocardial infarction follows a sudden cessation of blood supply to part of the myocardium of the left ventricle, resulting in necrosis of the ischaemic tissue, and eventual replacement by a fibrous scar. The classical presentation of myocardial infarction (MI) is similar to that of angina, except that the episode of chest pain is prolonged (usually more than 30 min), is not relieved by GTN and is associated with sweating, pallor, breathlessness, nausea and palpitation. In a minority of elderly patients, the presentation is atypical with confusion, syncope or breathlessness, but no chest pain. The immediate mortality is 30% in the 4 weeks following infarction and chiefly occurrs in the first 2 hr after the event. If an MI is suspected, the patient should be given a soluble aspirin (this has been shown to improve long-term survival) and a rapid referral to hospital for monitoring in a Coronary Care Unit. Speed of response is crucial because of the high early mortality caused by arrhythmias. Age should be no barrier to access to these facilities.

Heart failure

Heart failure is the single commonest cause of death in persons over 65 years. Cardiac failure is defined as the inability of the heart to pump blood adequately to meet the body's requirements, and in the elderly is most often due to failure of the myocardium. It may present acutely from a sudden deterioration of left ventricular function with marked distress and breathlessness, cough productive of pink frothy sputum (pulmonary oedema), cyanosis and peripheral vasoconstriction. Acute heart failure is managed by sitting the patient upright, administering oxygen, and giving intravenous morphine and frusemide. Chronic heart failure is managed with diuretics and angiotensin converting enzyme (ACE) inhibitors.

Chronic rheumatic heart disease

Valvular heart disease may occur following acute rheumatic fever in childhood, and is not uncommon in the elderly. The mitral valve is the most commonly affected. Patients may present with complaints of breathlessness, palpitations, recurrent bronchitis or fatigue. Complications include heart failure, systemic embolism and subacute infective endocarditis. Prophylactic amoxycillin (or erythromycin) should be given before any local dental treatment, because of the risk of endocarditis which has a 30% mortality rate in the elderly.

Excellent results can be achieved with cardiac surgery in elderly patients. Age alone is not now recognised as diminishing the benefits that can result from appropriate surgical treatment.

Diabetes mellitus

Diagnosis

Diabetes mellitus is an important cause of morbidity and mortality in old age. Impaired carbohydrate tolerance appears to be a normal feature of ageing, as both fasting and mean blood glucose concentration rise with increasing age. However, an elderly patient with typical symptoms of diabetes and a random blood glucose concentration of >11.1 mmol/l, or a fasting one of 7.8 mmol/l should be considered to have the condition.

Prevalence and presentation

The incidence of diabetes mellitus rises with age, with a 3% prevalence in those over 65 years of age. The majority are obese and non-insulin dependent. There is a wide spectrum of clinical presentation of diabetes mellitus in the elderly. Many asymptomatic patients are detected on routine urine or blood testing. Some have symptoms referable to diabetes, particularly thirst, weight loss and polyuria. Others present with an infection, and candidal vulvo-vaginitis is often the first indication of diabetes.

Complications

Vascular disease

Coronary heart disease, cerebrovascular disease and peripheral vascular disease are responsible for much of the increased morbidity and mortality in elderly patients with diabetes mellitus.

Diabetes also produces changes in small blood vessels, the most important being thickening of the capillary basement membrane. These changes are particularly relevant in the renal glomeruli and in the retina.

Peripheral neuropathy

One of the most serious complications of diabetes is peripheral nerve degeneration in the lower extremities. This is a direct consequence of poor metabolic control of diabetes. A number of patterns of diabetic neuropathy are recognised, some of which cause painful paraesthesiae, loss of sensation and wasting of the small muscles of the foot.

A common and serious consequence is ulceration and infection of the neuropathic diabetic foot resulting from reduced pain sensation. The lesion often begins with a small painless cut, but expands to form an extensive area of infection, necrosis and ulceration, progressing to gangrene, septicaemia and amputation (**30**).

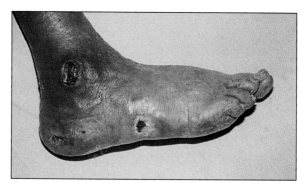

30 Diabetic foot ulcer.

Renal disease

Small vessel disease of the kidneys of diabetic patients gives rise to problems of proteinuria and renal failure. Diabetic nephropathy is related to the duration of the disease.

Vision

Diabetes mellitus affects the vision by the formation of premature cataract and the condition of retinopathy. The quality of blood glucose control has a key influence on the incidence and progression of diabetic eye disease. One in 10 patients with diabetes over the age of 60 years have retinopathy at the time of diagnosis. Elderly diabetic patients undergo regular ophthalmological testing to ensure adequate assessment and treatment.

Infections

Diabetic patients have an increased susceptibility to infection owing to impaired lymphocyte function. The effects of ageing and diabetes together may mask many features of infection such as pyrexia, leucocytosis and focal signs and the condition may go unrecognized.

Acute metabolic imbalance

Diabetic ketoacidosis is common in young diabetics with insulin-dependent diabetes. However, although less common in the elderly, the condition has a high mortality rate.

Management

The aims of management of diabetes in the elderly are to achieve relief from symptoms of hyperglycaemia, while avoiding hypoglycaemia and complications where possible. However, care must be taken to ensure that the prevention of long-term complications are not achieved at the expense of convenience of patients with a limited life expectancy. There may also be problems of ensuring compliance with treatment in mentally and physically frail individuals.

Diet and oral hypoglycaemic drugs are the mainstay of treatment aiming to achieve normoglycaemia and to minimize complications. Many elderly diabetics carry out their own monitoring by testing either urine or blood.

Cerebrovascular disease

Definitions

A stroke (or cerebrovascular accident) is a sudden interruption of the blood flow. Precise clinical features depend upon the localisation and extent of the brain damage. About 80% of strokes are due to cerebral infarction, and about 15% are due to haemorrhage (**31**). Transient Ischaemic Attacks (TIAs) are episodes of focal cerebral disturbance of rapid onset, and have a duration of less than 24 hours, with complete resolution. The importance of TIAs is that they may be an indication of an impending full-blown stroke.

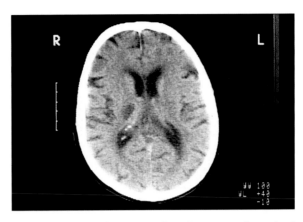

31 Computerized tomography (CT) scan of cerebral infarction of internal capsule (stroke).

Epidemiology

Stroke is the third major killer (after heart disease and cancer) in Western society and is the major cause of disability. The incidence of stroke increases with advancing age. Hypertension, heart disease, glucose intolerance, obesity, raised serum cholesterol and cigarette smoking all contribute to stroke. Cerebrovascular disease is the commonest cause of epilepsy in old age, and many patients require anticonvulsant therapy after a stroke.

Clinical features

The most obvious feature of a stroke is the weakness that affects one side of the body. Muscle tone is also affected, with hypertonia occurring in 15–59% of stroke patients, and hypotonia in 12–68%, depending on the time of examination following the stroke. Spasticity, if not controlled in the early stages, leads to permanent flexion deformity; persistent flaccidity is associated with a poor outcome as patients cannot control a limb if it has no muscle tone (**32**). Sensory problems related to cortical damage are major barriers to recovery, as the perception of what is to be carried out and why, is affected. Patients with these problems are at best clumsy, and at worst oblivious to the existence of one-half of their body, and may even deny their illness. Speech may be impaired following a stroke if there is damage in the receptive cortex of the parietotemporal area (Wernicke's area) or the frontal lobe (Broca's area). The former leaves the patient unable to understand instructions (receptive dysphasia) and the latter leaves an impediment in

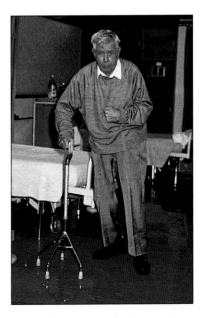

32 Stroke patient with characteristic flexed posture.

the production of speech (expressive dysphasia). Elements of both receptive and expressive dysphasias may occur in the same patient.

Emotional control is as much a function of the brain as is speech or motor power, and although emotional reactions appear spontaneous, we do in fact keep a very tight control over them. This control can be lost in a stroke and cause emotional lability, in which the patient readily bursts into tears or laughs excessively. An overly sympathetic response to such an outburst will merely exacerbate it, so it is better simply to ignore it.

Management

Hospital admission is usually required to confirm the diagnosis, to prevent and limit complications and to provide rehabilitation care. Not all stroke patients have the potential to benefit from a rehabilitation programme. Those with poor prospects for recovery include those experiencing severe loss of motor power, sensory loss, dysphasia and urinary or faecal incontinence.

Rehabilitation

Most recovery takes place during the first 6 months following the stroke, and patients with good potential will be cared for in a rehabilitation unit (**33**).

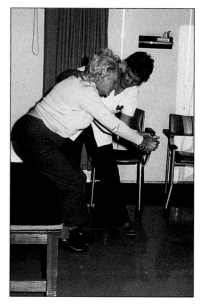

33 Stroke patient undergoing rehabilitation.

Parkinson's disease

Parkinson's disease is the commonest disabling neurological condition after stroke and affects 1–3% of the elderly population. It is a disorder of voluntary motor function.

Aetiology

Idiopathic Parkinson's disease is of unknown aetiology, although current theories have identified a genetic component. A syndrome discovered in opioid abusers exposed to the chemical MPTP closely resembles Parkinson's disease, and strongly raises the possibility of an aetiological role of an environmental toxin.

Secondary Parkinsonism may be drug-induced, most often as a side-effect of treatment with major tranquillisers of the phenothiazine group (chlorpromazine or prochlorperazine) or butyrophenones (such as haloperidol).

Pathology

The main pathological changes are extensive dopaminergic neuronal degeneration in the substantia nigra and locus coruleus, and the appearance of Lewy bodies (hyaline eosinophilic inclusion bodies) in the nerve cells in these areas. There is an overlap between the changes of Parkinsonism, normal ageing and Alzheimer's disease.

Clinical features

The symptoms are rigidity, tremor (pill-rolling) of the hands, feet, or head, and bradykinesia (slow movement). The classical picture is of immobile flexion at all joints, and a shuffling gait, with an absence of the normal arm swing (**34**). The face is expressionless and unblinking (**35**), and the speech quiet (dysphonia), monotonous and often slurred. In long-standing cases, there may be difficulty in initiating movement (rising from a chair), poor balance with frequent falls, and characteristic small handwriting (micrographia). Tremor is often the most distressing symptom, causing profound social embarrassment, making eating and drinking difficult, and worsened by anxiety. Swallowing difficulties may arise, producing drooling of saliva.

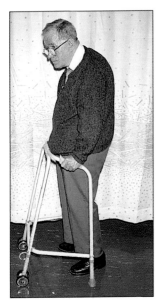

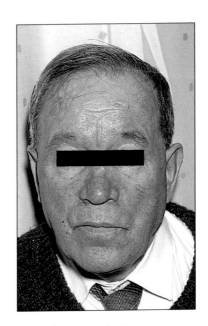

34 Parkinson's disease patient with characteristic stooped posture.

35 Parkinsonian facies.

Treatment

Severe depletion of the neurotransmitter dopamine was discovered in 1960 in the substantia nigra of Parkinson's patients, and so the combination of levodopa with peripheral dopa-decarboxylase inhibitors (Madopar or Sinemet) is now the mainstay of treatment for the majority of patients. Unfortunately, levodopa has no effect on the progression of the disease, and one in six patients fail to respond to it. Of those who respond initially, more than one-third lose this response in 3–5 years. For this reason, most doctors commence treatment only when the disease is producing significant disability. In addition to loss of efficacy, there are other problems of management in the later stages of Parkinson's disease. 'On-off' effect occurs with unpredictable swings in neurological performance, varying from good mobility to complete disability.

'Freezing episodes' occur when the mobile patient becomes suddenly stuck to the ground for a period of time. Involuntary movements, hallucinations, dizziness and delirium may all occur.

Selegiline is a selective MAOB-inhibitor that acts by inhibiting degradation of dopamine in the central nervous system. It may delay progression of the disease by exerting a neuroprotective role; for this reason and its levodopa-sparing effects, its use is recommended by some doctors early in the treatment of Parkinson's disease.

Transplantation of fetal brain tissue for the treatment of Parkinson's disease has received much publicity, but the results have proved disappointing. Considerable ethical and technical problems remain to be resolved, and at present this form of treatment should be regarded as experimental only.

Dementias

Primary dementias

Dementia is a syndrome characterised by an acquired global deterioration of the functions of the brain including intellect, memory and personality. Between 3% and 14% of people over the age of 65 years suffer from a dementing syndrome. There is a progressive rise in incidence with increasing age, from only 2% of those aged 65–69 years with evidence of dementia, to 22% of those aged 80 years and over.

The early symptoms tend to be ill-defined. Relatives may notice that the patient is becoming forgetful, losing things, missing appointments and becoming dependent on written lists to complete even the simplest of tasks. As the disease progresses sufferers are restless by day, and may wander disorientated at night. Sufferers may literally be unable to remember an instruction from one minute to the next, although often a good social facade is preserved. Demented patients become moody, angry and aggressive and tasks that would before have been dealt with easily prove baffling. Gradually, in the late stages of the condition, personal hygiene and social skills deteriorate and the patient becomes unable to dress or wash unaided and incontinent of urine or faeces.

Many disorders can produce the syndrome of dementia. These include Alzheimer's disease, multi-infarct dementia, Huntington's disease, Pick's disease, Parkinson's disease and even AIDS. In the elderly, however, three main conditions result in dementia, namely Alzheimer's disease, multi-infarct dementia and mixed dementia resulting from a combination of the first two.

Alzheimer's disease (AD) is the commonest type of dementia in the elderly, and the clinical course is one of relentless and progressive decline. The condition cannot be diagnosed with certainty during life, but at post mortem senile plaques with an amyloid core and neurofibrillary tangles occur most prominently in the hippocampus and cerebral cortex. Like Parkinson's disease, deficiency of a neurotransmitter, in this case acetylcholine has been identified in AD. A variety of drugs have been developed to enhance the functioning of the cholinergic system, in the hope of treating AD, but none have been particularly successful.

After AD, multi-infarct dementia (MID) is the commonest type of dementia in the elderly. It is caused by several strokes or infarcts. These destroy small areas of cells, impairing the blood supply. The strokes may be so slight that they are not noticed at the time. MID is hard to differentiate from AD during life, but clues to a diagnosis of MID include an abrupt onset with a step-wise deterioration and fluctuating course, and a history of strokes or hypertension. High blood pressure, smoking, alcohol and a family history are all risk factors for MID. Many of these factors can be modified and, as people adopt healthier lifestyles, the incidence of stroke is declining.

Most demented people, particularly those with mild dementia, can continue to live in the community with assistance from relatives and social and health services. Institutional care may become necessary when problems of immobility, incontinence or behavioural disturbance occurs. The decision to seek institutional care can be a difficult one, with care-givers feeling a desire for relief after years of strain, yet regarding the necessity to institutionalise their relative as a sign of failure.

Symptoms like anxiety, agitation and paranoia are best treated with a low dose of phenothiazine, for example thioridazine. Time and tolerance are the best tools in the management of dementia. Simple practice and rehearsal of skills and actions may cause them to reappear. Benefit can be derived by encouraging emotional memories as well as cognitive skills as exemplified by 'reality orientation' and 'reminiscence' therapies.

Secondary dementias

In a small percentage of cases, dementia is a secondary phenomenon to an underlying medical condition, for example hypothyroidism, vitamin B_{12} deficiency, subdural haematoma or drug toxicity. Treatment of the primary condition will result in resolution of the dementia, so failure to recognise and treat a secondary dementia is a tragedy for the patient.

Acute confusional states

Although dementia is generally an irreversible condition involving progressive deterioration, an acute confusional state is a temporary period of cognitive impairment and lasts only a matter of days or weeks. It often occurs when an old person is suffering a major physical illness, which may not necessarily directly involve the brain. Indeed, the onset of an acute confusional state is often the first sign of major illness in an elderly person. Many factors can produce delirium. These include drug toxicity, infection, heart failure and disseminated malignancy. An acute confusional state is characterised by rapid onset, with clouded consciousness, disorientation and impairment of memory, slurred and disjointed speech and disturbed perception, often resulting in hallucinations. The serious nature of the acute confusional state is evidenced by studies showing a 23% death rate in patients presenting in this way. Recognition of the condition is important to facilitate prompt treatment of the underlying medical disorder.

Osteoarthritis

Two-thirds of people aged 65 years and over suffer from the symptoms of osteoarthritis. Radiological evidence of the condition is present in 90% of this group.

Pathophysiology

Osteoarthritis represents a failure of joint function resulting from the interaction of mechanical and environmental conditions. The primary damage is to the articular cartilage which becomes less elastic and splits into fissures. Overgrowth of surrounding bone occurs.

Clinical features

The joints most commonly involved are the hips, knees, lumbosacral and cervical spine, and proximal and distal interphalangeal (**36**). Symptoms include pain and stiffness of the affected joints, characteristically relieved by rest and worst at the end of the day. As the disease progresses, joint deformity and instability occurs, Joint movement is painful and restricted and the muscles that move the joint gradually waste.

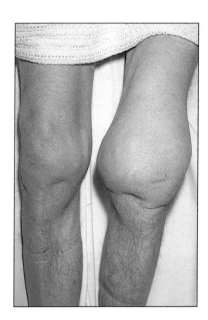

36 Osteoarthritis of knees.

Treatment

Simple measures such as weight reduction, physiotherapy and other exercise can strengthen the muscles around affected joints and preserve a good range of movement. First line drug treatment would include the use of a simple analgesic like paracetamol, which is very effective in both relieving pain and reducing inflammation. If this approach has failed, then a non-steroidal anti-inflammatory drug (NSAID) like ibuprofen may be tried. However, the NSAIDs are notoriously poorly tolerated in the elderly, frequently causing gastrointestinal haemorrhage, fluid retention or

Table 10. Patients most at risk from NSAIDs.

1. The elderly
2. Multiple drug use
3. Increased NSAID dose
4. Increased NSAID duration
5. Impaired renal function
6. Coexisting collagen disorders

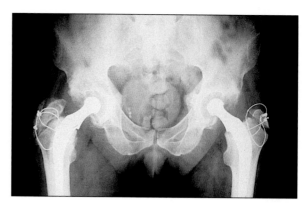

37 X-ray of bilateral prosthetic hips (Charnley).

renal damage, and must always be used with great caution (**Table 10**). Joint replacement surgery represents the greatest single advance in the treatment of arthritis this century. Joint replacement is most useful for patients with refractory pain in a single joint or with only one severely affected joint (**37**). The success rate in relieving pain is high (90% or greater). There is no upper age limit on suitability of patient for this operation.

Osteoporosis

The pathological definition of osteoporosis is a decreased amount of bone. Anatomically, the bone is of normal dimensions, but contains less bone tissue per unit volume. An osteoporotic bone is weaker than average, and the importance of the condition lies in its predisposing to fractures. The three main fracture sites associated with osteoporosis are hip (proximal femur), wrist (distal forearm) and back (vertebral bodies). Such fractures produce considerable pain and disability and an example of this is the fact that one third of patients fracturing their hip die within 6 months and those who survive, half will suffer pain or increased dependency (**38**).

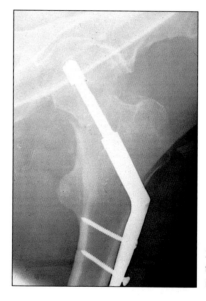

38 X-ray of fractured hip with nail inserted.

Pathogenesis

Osteoporosis is a complex disorder with multiple causes, and the main cause of age-related fractures is a low bone density. Bone density depends on two variables: the amount of bone made during growth (peak bone mass) and its subsequent rate of loss. The menopause produces an accelerated phase of bone loss that lasts up to 10 years and this is the basis for use of hormone replacement therapy (HRT) in menopausal women. Those women at greatest risk of osteoporosis are thin, with a strong family history of the condition, physically inactive, cigarette smokers, with an inadequate dietary intake of calcium.

Clinical features

Osteoporosis may declare itself, by the fracture of a long bone following minimal trauma, as an episode of severe back pain with vertebral collapse, or simply a shortening of the trunk height, often passing unnoticed by patient and family. The wedge-shaped collapse of vertebral bodies results in a fixed forward flexion of the spine, producing a kyphosis (**39**). Vertebral fracture or collapse often occurs spontaneously producing sudden onset of severe back pain. The fracture may render the patient bed-bound with pain, which settles over a period of 4–5 weeks.

Treatment

Calcium

Although dietary calcium supplements are widely used in the prevention and treatment of osteoporosis, there is considerable disagreement about their role. The elderly may take a diet deficient in calcium and this, together with an age-related decrease in intestinal absorption and increased urinary excretion of calcium, is a persuasive argument for its use. A daily calcium intake of 1500 mg calcium has been shown to reduce the rate of cortical bone loss in established osteoporosis, but there is no clear evidence of subsequent reduction in fracture rate.

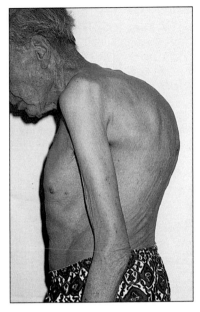

39 Lateral view of osteoporotic kyphosis.

Exercise

Load-bearing is an important mechanical stimulus to the skeleton, as bone cells respond to mechanical stresses and strains. Immobilisation results in considerable bone loss, due to both a reduction in bone formation and an increase in resorption. Clear evidence exists that weight-wearing exercise in the elderly can decrease the rate of bone loss, and benefit the skeleton. Beneficial effects on muscle bulk may also improve tone and balance, and may act as a splint in the event of a fall.

Drugs in the elderly

The extent of drug prescribing in the elderly is an important issue that has, in recent years, received considerable attention. Prescribing rates for the elderly continue to rise, compared with a slight fall in other age groups. It is estimated that 39% of the entire NHS drugs bill is consumed in prescriptions for the elderly who constitute only 17% of the population. Studies indicate that 80% of old people admitted to hospital are prescribed at least one drug per day, and as many as 25% are taking four to six daily. In addition, adverse reactions to drugs are implicated, at least in part, in 10% of all elderly hospital admissions

Polypharmacy

Polypharmacy means the prescription of more than one drug simultaneously. This is the norm in old age, with some unfortunate elderly subjects taking as many as nine different drugs every day

(**40**). The phenomenon of polypharmacy has arisen partly from repeat prescribing, and partly from awareness of multiple pathology and a desire to alleviate the many disabilities from which old people suffer. It is even possible for the unwary practitioner to spiral disastrously into the prescription of drugs to counteract the side-effects of those already prescribed. Around 36% of old people are also taking over-the-counter (OTC) medication, of which their own doctors are unaware, which exacerbates the problem.

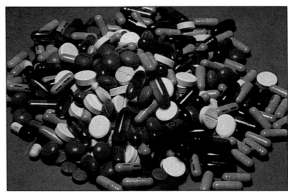

40 Array of multiple tablets (compliance).

Adverse drug reactions (ADRs)

Definition: 'Any response to a drug that is noxious and unintended, and which occurs at doses used in man for prophylaxis, diagnosis or treatment.'

It has been suggested that ADRs are the inevitable price we pay for the benefits of modern drug therapy. The susceptibility of the elderly to ADRs has been well established, and increasing age is an important predictive factor for an ADR in patients admitted to hospital. The overall incidence is two to three times that found in young adults. Furthermore, the incidence is underestimated because ADRs are less readily recognised by the elderly themselves, and because the reactions may mimic the characteristics of disease states.

Factors influencing susceptibility to ADRs

Polypharmacy

It has been clearly demonstrated that the incidence of ADRs increases with the number of drugs taken. The incidence of ADRs increases exponentially rather than linearly with the number of drugs given to patients, indicating that the effects of multiple drugs use is not merely additive.

Type of drug

In many cases those drugs with a low therapeutic index, such as digoxin and warfarin. Other commonly implicated drugs include diuretics, NSAIDs, theophylline and benzodiazepines.

Pharmacological factors

The majority of ADRs are dose related. The pharmacokinetic process is concerned with the absorption, distribution and elimination of drugs, and can be studied by measurement of drug concentration in the blood or urine. Age-related alterations in the pharmacokinetic process result in higher serum and tissue concentrations in the elderly, which may lead to a higher incidence of ADRs (**Table 11**).
1. Absorption. Age produces little effect on the absorption of drugs.

Table 11. Changes in drug handling in the elderly.

1. Absorption	Essentially unchanged
2. Distribution	Lipid-soluble drugs prolonged action water-soluble drugs increased risk of toxicity
3. Metabolism	Little effect
4. Excretion	Glomerular filtration and tubular secretion rates decline. Dose reduction necessary in drugs with predominant renal elimination.

2. Distribution. The distribution of a drug in the body depends on body composition, plasma-protein binding and blood flow to the individual organs. With age, there is a relative decrease in total body water and lean body mass and an increase in body fat. Lipid-soluble drugs, like diazepam, have an increased volume of distribution, which results in prolonged action because of longer elimination half-lives. Conversely, the volume of distribution of water-soluble drugs like ethanol and digoxin is reduced, thereby increasing the peak plasma concentration for a given dose, and hence the risk of toxicity.

3. Metabolism. The clearance of drugs by the liver depends on the activity of the enzymes responsible for biotransformation and on liver blood flow. Hepatic blood flow alters little with age, and minor changes in drug-metabolizing capacity with age are thought to have little influence on drug toxicity.

4. Excretion. The best documented alteration in pharmacokinetics with age is the reduction in the rate of elimination of drugs by the kidneys. Both the glomerular filtration and tubular secretion rates decline with age. Drugs with predominantly renal elimination and potentially toxic effects in the elderly include digoxin, cimetidine, lithium, NSAIDs and the aminoglycoside antibiotics. The doses of all of these drugs may require reduction in the elderly.

5. Pharmacodynamics. The pharmacodynamic process include the pharmacological effects that are responsible for the eventual therapeutic effect and also those responsible for the adverse effects. Generalisations are difficult, and the effect of age on sensitivity to drug varies with the drug studied and the response measured. In some cases the responsiveness is increased and the elderly are more sensitive to pharmacological effects, so the dose must be decreased, for example with the benzodiazepines and warfarin. In other cases, for example, with beta-adrenergic drugs, the response is decreased.

Hoarding

Hoarding of drugs can easily follow multiple prescribing and form a misplaced sense of thriftiness on the part of the patient. This is not a problem confined to the elderly. Some drugs lose their effectiveness if stored for prolonged periods, e.g. glyceryl trinitrate tablets, and patients may inadvertently take hoarded drugs for the wrong indications.

Compliance

Definition: 'Compliance is the extent to which the patients behaviour coincides with the clinical prescription.'

It is now widely acknowledged that non-adherence to prescription is widespread, and certainly not a problem exclusive to the elderly. Estimates of non-compliance vary, but 75% of older patients make errors in taking their medication, one-quarter of which are considered to be serious. In the elderly the difficulty may be aggravated by poor memory, poor vision and hearing, difficulty opening containers and having to cope with dosage regimes that would tax much younger patients (**40, 41**). Compliance may be optimized by counselling patients about their drugs, and by providing clear written instructions on a separate card. Those most at risk of poor compliance are those over 85 years, living alone, receiving multiple drugs, with a long duration of treatment, and psychiatric problems or cognitive impairment. Assistance with medication may be sought from a spouse, carer or district nurse who will supervise the administration of treatment.

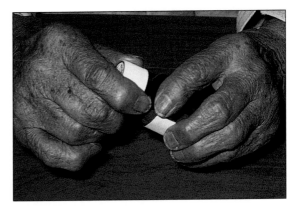

41 Arthritic hands attempting to open bottle (compliance).

There is little point in prescribing for those with severe memory problems unless steps are taken to ensure supervision by a third party. The more detailed information provided on a prescription, the better the compliance. Drug, dose, time to be taken and special instructions, e.g. before food, must all be included. Unless specified, all prescriptions will be supplied in a child-proof container. Drugs affecting the mouth are described in **Table 12**.

Table 12. Drugs affecting the mouth.

1. Xerostomia	Anticholinergic drugs e.g. tricyclic antidepressants. Also levodopa, phenothiazines and antihistamines.
2. Taste disturbance	Penicillamine, metronidazole.
3. Hypersensitivity reactions	
Type I (immediate)	e.g. lignocaine, mepivacaine.
Type II (delayed)	e.g. phenolphthalein, tetracycline, gold, indomethacin, captopril.
Erythema multiforme (mouth, eye and urogenital ulceration)	e.g. sulphonamides, barbiturates, penicillin.
4. Oral ulceration	Aspirin, potassium, anti-neoplastic agents.
5. Gingival hypertrophy	Phenytoin.
6. Discoloration of oral mucosa and teeth	Lead, chlorpromazine, tetracycline.
7. Oral infections	Corticosteroids, antibiotics, immunosuppressive drugs.
8. Extrapyramidal syndromes	Orofacial dyskinesia e.g. phenothiazines, levodopa.
9. Drug-induced blood dyscrasias	Suspect if spontaneous bleeding, pallor of oral mucosa, unresponsive oral infections, easy bruising, ulcerated mucosa and pyrexia e.g. chloramphenicol, sulphonamides, phenytoin, gold, penicillamine, phenothiazines, tricyclic antidepressants.

History relevant to drug treatment

Enquiry should concentrate on present or past medical conditions that may be affected by your treatment.

1. Cardiovascular disease. Enquire about heart problems, angina, heart attacks, episodic loss of consciousness and undue breathlessness on exertion.
2. Respiratory disease. Enquire about smoking habits, exercise tolerance, and chronic wheeze or cough. Patients who are unable to dress without pausing to get their breath back are likely to be suffering severe lung disease.

   Patients with chronic obstructive airways disease may be dependent on hypoxic drive as the main stimulus to respiration. Great caution should be taken with the administration of oxygen to elderly patients with chronic lung disease, as a respiratory arrest may be precipitated.
3. Other medical conditions. Specific enquiry about diabetes mellitus, epilepsy and rheumatic heart disease should be made.
4. Bleeding tendencies. Enquire about recent bleeding episodes, for example nose bleeds and easy bruising. Affirmative answers may prompt you to postpone treatment until appropriate investigations have been undertaken.
5. Present drug therapy. Ideally, patients should be required to bring all present medication to each consultation with the dentist. Some patients may produce a written list of medications. Specific enquiry should be made about whether the patient is taking steroid or warfarin therapy. If there is any doubt about medication, the patients general medical practitioner should be contacted. The greatest hazard with diabetic patients is unnoticed hypoglycaemia and hypoglycaemic agents should never be given to patients who are fasting.
6. Home circumstances. If you are initiating therapy

in a frail elderly patient, it is prudent to check who will take the prescription to the chemist and who will supervise medication. The carer or home help can usually undertake this function.

Rational prescribing for the elderly

1. Accurate diagnosis. Care in diagnosis, requiring accuracy, and based on a knowledge of modified presentation in the elderly, and a firm clinical indication before starting a course of drug treatment.
2. Drug regime. A simple but effective policy measure is to ensure that at every consultation, the patient is required to bring all drug supplies along to show the dentist. Prescribe the minimum number of drugs together with the simplest possible regime, attempting to use the same time schedule if possible.
3. Drug formulation. Most drugs are available in a variety of formulations including tablets, capsules, elixirs, soluble and parenteral preparations. There is an age-related reduction in oesophageal motility which increases the hazard from irritant substances and capsules, which may lodge in the oesophagus and cause painful spasms, stricture or even perforation. The risk is reduced by either prescribing a liquid formulation or advising the patient to take his medication with a full glass of water, seated in the upright position. In addition, patients who have cerebrovascular or Parkinson's disease may suffer from difficulty in swallowing, and a selection of a soluble preparation may be appropriate.
4. Presentation. Clear packaging, labelling and instructions are essential.
5. Dose. Use an appropriate dose regime, starting with the minimum effective dose adjusted, where indicated, by knowledge of pharmacokinetic and pharmacodynamic changes with age.
6. Adverse effects. Always be alert to the possibility of drug-induced illness, and always consider drugs as the cause of any acute confusional state.
7. Review. Define the intended duration of treatment, supported by an automatic mechanism for review or withdrawal.

A policy for managing pain relief is described in Table 13.

Table 13. Managing pain relief.

1. Identify the cause.	Jaw pain due to angina pectoris will not respond to paracetamol, but should be treated with sublingual glyceryl trinitrate tablets or spray.
2. Provide adequate dosage.	Successful analgesia is prescribed regularly in anticipation of the pain.
3. Consider adjunctive measures.	Laxatives should be co-prescribed with opiates, and antidepressants may act as an effective adjunct to analgesia with trigeminal neuralgia.
4. Use a scaled approach.	Decide whether the pain is mild, moderate or severe, and select your analgesic accordingly.
Mild pain	Paracetamol
Moderate pain	Coproxamol codydramol, nefopam hydrochloride
Severe pain	Morphine, diamorphine

Further reading

Andrews, K. 1987. *Rehabilitation of the Older Adult.* Edward Arnold, Sevenoaks.

Coni, N., Davison, W. & Webster, S. 1988. *Lecture Notes on Geriatrics.* Blackwell Scientific Publications, Oxford.

Davies, D.M. (ed.). 1985. *Textbook of Adverse Drug Reactions.* Oxford Medical, Oxford.

Denham, M.J. & George, C.F. (eds). 1990. Drugs in Old Age. New Perspectives. *British Medical Bulletin* **46**(1), 1–299.

Hildick-Smith, M. (ed.). 1985. *Neurological Problems in Old Age.* Baillière Tindall, London.

Jorm, A.F. 1987. *Understanding Senile Dementia.* Croom Helm, London.

Mace, N.L. & Rabins, P.V. 1981. *The 36 Hour Day.* Warner Books.

MacLennan, W.J. & Peden, N.R. 1989. *Metabolic and Endocrine Problems in the Elderly.* Springer-Verlag, Berlin.

Smith, R. (ed.). 1990. *Osteoporosis 1990.* Royal College of Physicians of London, London.

4. The Ageing Mouth

A number of age changes affecting the orofacial structures are of clinical importance when caring for elderly dental patients and some of these changes will make certain clinical procedures more difficult and limit the prognosis of treatment. This is particularly true in prosthetic and restorative treatment. Other oral age changes need to be recognized by the dental surgeon as being normal and not part of a disease process. Considerable reassurance can be given to the older and worried patient if the dentist is familiar with these changes.

Dental tissues

The enamel, dentine, cementum and pulp tissue all undergo a number of well-recognised changes with age. Many of the changes encountered are not age changes *per se* but are as a result of the incremental effects of wear, disease and habit (see Chapters 6, 7, 9 and 10) (**42**).

One important change, of clinical significance, is the gradual increase in enamel surface fluoride with age. As well as altering the resistance to caries attack, the increased surface fluoride reduces the ability of phosphoric acid to etch enamel when composite restorations are being placed.

Changes that occur in the dentine pulp complex are familiar to all dentists because of the clinical effects these changes have. The dentine becomes more sclerotic and less elastic. Deposition of secondary and reparative (tertiary) dentine is particularly prominent on the ceiling and floor of the pulp chamber, but less so on the walls (**43**). These changes may lead to a reduction in the dentinal sensitivity in elderly patients. In addition to a reduction in the volume of the pulp chamber, there is an increased incidence of pulpal calcification in the elderly. This may be diffuse, or in the form of

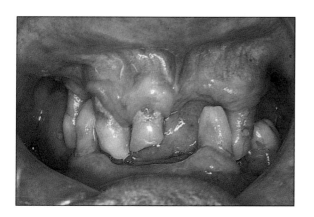

42 The dentition of an elderly patient showing the effects of dental disease as opposed to specific age changes.

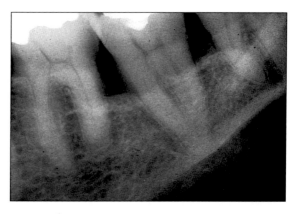

43 Radiograph of $\overline{67}$ showing reduction in the dimensions of pulp chambers in heavily restored elderly teeth.

pulp stones, and is related to previous dentinal and/or pulpal injury. Reparative dentine may be laid down over the orifices to root canals and a generalised narrowing occurs along the full length of the canal, making root canal treatment difficult, but obliteration of the canal space is rare (see Chapter 7) (**44**).

Cementum thickness is directly proportional to age: the older the individual, the greater the thickness of cementum. Lateral and accessory canals slowly become obliterated, with the width of the apical foramina being gradually reduced. However, as long as vital pulp tissue remains, complete closure will not occur (**45**). The progressive age-related laying down of cementum should not be confused with hypercementosis or cemental tumours, which are pathological processes.

Atrophy is characteristic of the older pulp, with a decrease in the number and size of the cell population; however, there is an increase in the number of collagenous fibres, particularly in the coronal area, in old individuals. Blood vessels in the aged pulp also show a decrease in number and exhibit arteriosclerotic changes with reduced blood supply. This diminished blood supply probably renders the pulp more susceptible to irreversible injury. There is also a reduction in the number of nerve fibres which, coupled with the increase in secondary dentine, has the effect of reducing sensitivity to environmental stimuli.

As more elderly people are likely to retain teeth later in life, changes in the dental tissues will become increasingly important factors to consider in the restoration of such teeth.

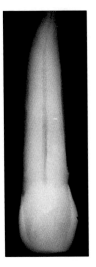

44 Radiograph of extracted tooth showing obliteration of pulp chamber and generalised narrowing of root canal.

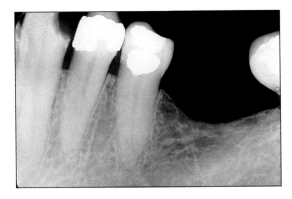

45 Radiograph of ⌐5 showing deposition of secondary cementum at apex with apical constriction approximately 3 mm from apex.

Periodontal tissues

It is important not to confuse age changes in periodontal tissues with those seen in disease processes (**46**). With disease the changes that occur in the periodontal tissue in young and old individuals are essentially the same (see Chapter 7) but there is some evidence to suggest an altered immune response in the elderly. With age there appears to be a reduction in the numbers of fibroblasts and the connective tissue fibres become coarse and less well organized. The periodontal membrane shows a decrease in width with age and it has been suggested that some of this reduction is caused by the continued deposition of cement at the root surface.

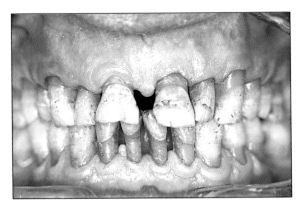

46 Dentition of an elderly patient with good oral hygiene and healthy periodontal tissue.

Oral mucosa

Changes in the skin and oral mucosa may lead to a number of problems. In the dermis of the skin there is a reduction in the collagen bundles and elastic content. Atrophic changes can also be found in the sebaceous and sweat glands and there is a reduction in the mean skin epithelial thickness with age.

Some initial oral changes may be noticed with the naked eye and these include sublingual varicosities (**373**), prominent sebaceous glands and a smooth appearance of some mucosal surfaces. Sublingual varicosities are found in many elderly individuals but their presence is not associated with cardiovascular disease and they should be regarded as a normal finding. There is also the impression that the mucosa is thinner and that underlying features, such as sebaceous glands, are more prominent, although epithelial proliferation rates are disputed. There is now good evidence that there is a reduction in mean epithelial thickness with age. In the tongue, a reduction of epithelial thickness of around one-third from young to old can be observed (**47**). Although the progenitor cell layer remains at a constant thickness, there is a reduction in the nuclear:cytoplasmic ratio. In addition, there is an overall simplification of the epithelial structure with age and the rete pegs become much less prominent.

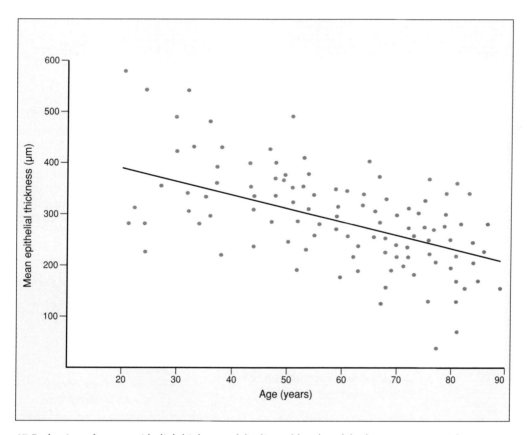

47 Reduction of mean epithelial thickness of the lingual border of the human tongue with age.

The epithelial surface of the tongue becomes smooth as filiform papillae are lost (**48**). In the circumvallate papillae, taste buds have been claimed to atrophy and to produce changes in the gustatory sensation. It had been suggested that a person aged 70 years has only 30% of the original complement of taste buds. However, more recent studies show that the number of taste buds does not decline with age and also that there is less change in taste thresholds than previously believed. Unlike taste acuity, there is considerable evidence for age-related declines in the sense of smell. Older people perceive certain stimuli as less intense than young individuals and perform less well in the identification of specific odours. Although there is some information about the structure of the epithelium in old individuals, little is known about functional variation with age, except that some histological changes would suggest that the mucosa is more easily damaged in the elderly.

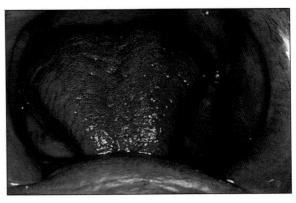

48 The characteristic appearance of the tongue and oral mucosa in an elderly individual.

Saliva and salivary glands

Saliva plays a central role in maintaining oral homeostasis. The combined secretions of all major and minor salivary glands produce 0.5–1.5 litres of saliva per day. Glandular saliva contains, besides water, many proteins with specific intra-oral actions and numerous electrolytes. Through these components, saliva protects all oral tissues, soft and hard, and facilitates the major functions of the mouth (alimentation and communication). A summary of the functional properties of saliva, and some key individual components mediating these functions, is shown in **Table 14**. Patients with disordered or diseased salivary glands provide clear examples of the necessary role that saliva plays in oral physiology. Salivary hypofunction can result in significant local and systemic consequences to the host, including rampant caries, candidiasis, dysphagia and considerable subjective discomfort (**Table 15**).

Table 14. Major functions of saliva.

Function	
Remineralization	Statherin, anionic proline-rich proteins
Anti-microbial	Secretory IgA, lysozyme, lactoferrin, lactoperoxidase, histatins, anti-HIV factor(s), mucin, amylase
Lubrication	Mucin, cationic proline-rich, glycoprotein, water
Digestion – food breakdown – food bolus formation/ translocation – gustation	 Amylase, proteases, DNase, RNase Mucin, water Water
Mucosal repair	Epidermal growth factor
Buffering capacity	Bicarbonate, phosphate, histatins

Table 15. Consequences of salivary hypofunction.

Rampant Caries
Candidiasis
Mucosal friability
Dysphagia
Complaints of oral dryness
Complaints of altered taste

Accordingly, early reports of marked reductions in salivary gland performance in elderly individuals was cause for significant concern, particularly since descriptive morphological studies showed parallel age-related changes in salivary parenchymal tissue. Modern studies of salivary gland structure and function date from about the mid-1970s. A key feature of the more recent investigations was an attempt to distinguish disease effects from ageing effects. For example, it was shown clearly and quantitatively by morphometric analyses that human major salivary glands show a relatively linear reduction in the proportional volume represented by acinar cells (**49**). This decrease is somewhat larger for the submandibular gland (~37%) than for parotid glands (~32%). Similar observations have been reported for minor salivary glands also, whose role in the maintenance of mucosal health may be of great importance (**50**, **51**). Importantly, these observations, although obtained with necropsy samples, were made on glands from individuals with negative histories for diseases or therapies known to affect salivary gland function. Consistent with these findings, a recent study showed a linear, age-associated decrease in computed tomographic (CT) density of parotid (**52**) and submandibular glands using CT scans with selected different-aged, living persons. Thus, it appears that physiological (i.e. disease-free) ageing is typically associated with diminished numbers of acinar cells in salivary

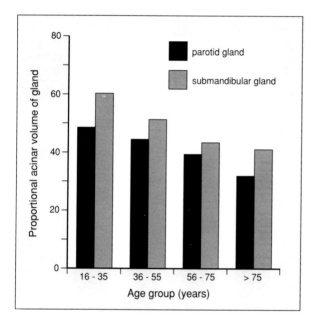

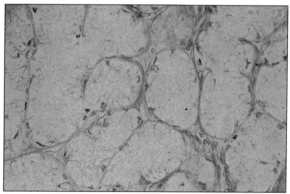

49 Proportional volume of acinar cells in parotid (filled) and submandibular (hatched) glands from different-aged individuals.

50 A minor salivary gland from a young individual showing close approximation of acinar elements.

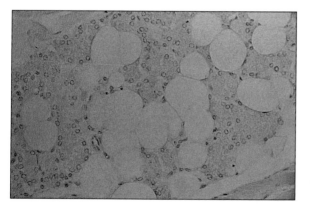

51 A minor serous salivary gland from an elderly individual showing adipose replacement. In the minor mucous glands, fibrous replacement is more prominent.

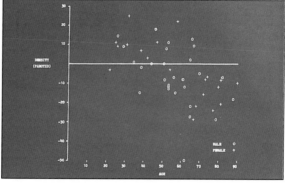

52 The X-ray density of the parotid glands in subjects of different ages.

glands. This is of special importance because acinar cells are the only cell type in the salivary glands capable of transporting fluid. Further, acinar cells make about 85–90% of the secreted proteins found in saliva with key oral functions (**Table 14**).

It would be reasonable to expect that this reduction in acinar cell mass would result in diminished salivary gland secretory performance (fluid output and exocrine protein release). However, this has not been observed and studies demonstrated no changes in citric acid-stimulated parotid flow rate in different-aged healthy individuals. This type of secretion (stimulated, **53**) mimics that experienced during alimentation. This cross-sectional ageing finding has been reproduced by others and a recently reported longitudinal study (same persons observed over a 10 year interval) of stimulated parotid function also showed no change in flow rates with age. In addition, a cross-sectional study of unstimulated (the basal secretion; primarily providing tissue protection) parotid flow rates indicated no functional alteration with increased age. While parotid output seems universally stable with healthy ageing, studies on submandibular flow rates have not been as consistent. These include a statistically significant reduction in this secretion among different-aged persons, and also no significant effect of age (**54**), despite some trends in that direction. Interestingly, submandibular gland secretion seems to be more vulnerable in various perturbations than parotid gland function (witness the dichotomous effects of Sjögren's syndrome and Alzheimer's disease on these two secretions).

It seems reasonable to suggest that if salivary flow rates decline with age, the declines are modest and may not affect all glands equally. Clinically significant diseases in flow rates and complaints of oral dryness in an older adult are not normal and should not be considered a natural consequence of growing old.

Several investigators have also examined exocrine protein secretion in parotid salivas from different-aged persons. In general, no significant

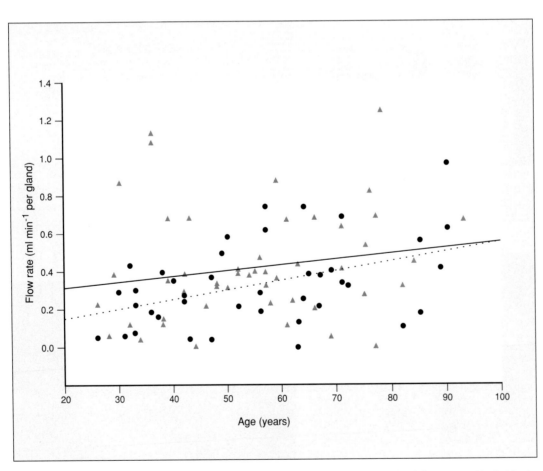

53 The distribution of 2% citrate-stimulated parotid salivary flow rates in healthy different-aged individuals: Δ, males; ○, females.

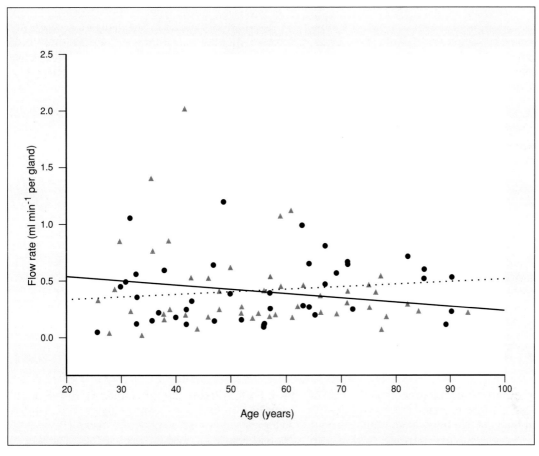

54 The distribution of 2% citrate-stimulated submandibular salivary flow rates in healthy different-aged individuals: Δ, males; O, females.

reductions between age groups have been observed (**55**) for a large number of individual components, including amylase, secretory IgA, anionic proline-rich proteins, lactoferrin and lysozyme.

What is the explanation for the failure of investigators to see any generally significant changes in salivary acinar cell functional measures (flow rate and exocrine protein release) despite the general occurrence of an age-associated reduced acinar cell volume in the salivary glands? Although not unequivocally supported, a possible explanation for these paradoxical findings has been suggested. It has been postulated that young adults have a substantial secretory reserve capacity (i.e. excess acinar tissue) which can be utilised (or drawn upon) later in life. This would mean that despite the loss of acinar tissue throughout the adult lifespan, normal (young-adult) levels of secretory function can be achieved, as long as there is no further stress on the system, i.e. an elderly person remains generally healthy. Most adults, however, are not free from disease. Although salivary hypofunction is not a

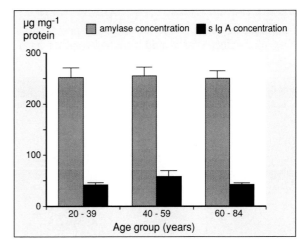

55 Content of amylase (hatched) and secretory IgA (shaded) in stimulated parotid saliva from different-aged persons. Values are mean ± SEM.

simple sequela of growing old, it is associated with many conditions (e.g. diseases, therapies) commonly observed in the elderly (**Table 16**). Thus, salivary glands of older persons may be viewed as endogenously adequately functional but vulnerable to external insults. In the presence of negative exogenous influences (such as anti-depressant drugs or X-radiation), perhaps the lack of a secretory reserve in elders renders the gland unable to function satisfactorily with the associated disastrous consequences referred to earlier (**Table 15**).

Table 16. Common conditions affecting salivary secretion in the elderly.

Condition	Examples
Medications	Antidepressants (eg. amitriptyline), Anticholingergics (eg. scopolamine), Antihypertensives (eg. clonidine)
Anti-neoplastic therapies	X-radiation, cytotoxic, chemotherapy, immunomodulatory chemotherapy
Autoimmune disease	Sjögren's syndrome

Muscle and nerve

A characteristic of the ageing process is the loss of muscle mass. There is evidence to suggest a reduction in total muscle mass amounting to about one-third over an 80-year period, with a still relatively larger annual loss when subjects of 70 and 80 years are compared. Electrophysiological studies of jaw-closing muscles have shown a prolongation of the contraction phase with age, indicating either a general age change of the muscle or the loss of faster twitch fibres (**56, 57**). However, consideration must be given to the fact that any preferential loss of one fibre type would have to be rather large to be identifiable using standard histological sampling techniques, and earlier electrophysiological studies have not shown discrete fibre type populations. It has been observed that grouping of fibre types does occur in certain arm and leg muscles of older subjects. Recent work on jaw muscles in the elderly has not shown signs of atrophy or a decrease in fast-contracting fibres.

In other studies it has been shown that there is a loss of motor units with age, particularly after the age of 60 years. These motor units in older subjects have longer contraction times (**58**) and exhibit a

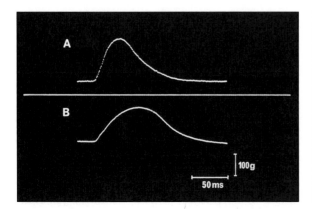

56 The averaged response of the masseter muscle in subjects of different age when stimulated to produce similar levels of twitch tension. Upper trace, young subject; lower trace, old subject.

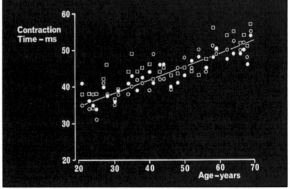

57 Contraction times of masseter muscles in subjects of different ages with three target forces for each individual.

reduction in their threshold firing rates (**59**), this being consistent with a more slowly contracting muscle developing a partly fused tetanic contraction at a lower frequency. There is also a significant reduction in maximum tension and in loss of isometric and dynamic muscle strength in older subjects. The cross-sectional area of a muscle is an important determinant of its maximum force and, using CT, it has been found that in two jaw-closing muscles, the masseter and medial pterygoid, there is a significant reduction of around 40% between the ages of 20 and 90 years (**60, 61, 62**). In all cases,

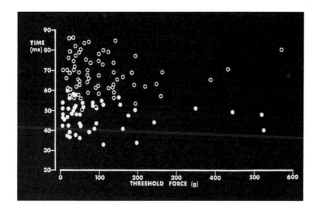

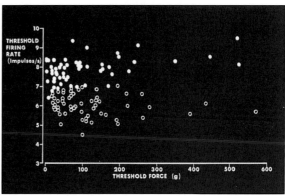

58 Contraction time of motor units in young and old individuals as a function of the force at which the units were recruited: ●, young subjects; O, old subjects.

59 Threshold firing rates of motor units in young and old individuals as a function of the force at which the units were recruited: ●, young subjects; O, old subjects.

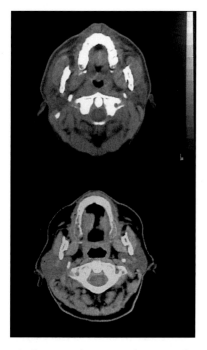

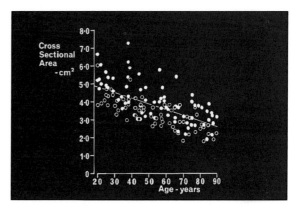

61 The cross-sectional area of the masseter muscle in subjects of different ages: ●, male; O, female.

60 Computed tomography scan of masseter and medial pterygoid muscles in a young and old individual. Upper trace, young subject; lower trace, old subject.

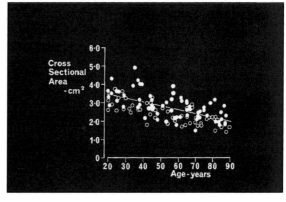

62 The cross-sectional area of the medial pterygoid muscle in subjects of different ages: ●, male; O, female.

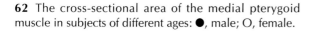

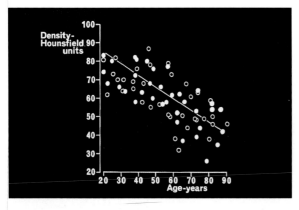

63 The X-ray density of the masseter muscle in subjects of different ages: ●, male; O, female.

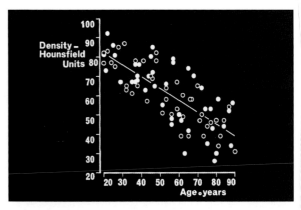

64 The X-ray density of the medial pterygoid muscle in subjects of different ages: ●, male; O, female.

female subjects exhibited significantly smaller muscles. In addition, changes in X-ray density of these muscles indicated an increase in the fibro-fatty content with increasing age (**63, 64**). These results are consistent with studies of the chest, abdomen, arm and leg muscles and may indicate a general age change of the muscle tissue in the body as a whole, and specifically a reduction in the masticatory forces that can be used by ageing subjects. Other work suggests that there is little variation in the average chewing cycle duration with age, perhaps supporting the notion of a central pattern generator for this function.

Superimposed on these changes, further reductions in jaw muscle bulk are found in edentulous subjects when compared with dentate subjects, supporting evidence that the level of masticatory force and chewing efficiency in patients where the natural dentition has been replaced by an artificial one is greatly reduced. It has also been reported that following a change in functional conditions, there appears to be a reduction in Type II fibres. In some patients it is considered appropriate to provide overdentures as part of their treatment (see Chapter 10) and, from recent work, it appears that their masticatory muscles have similar cross-sectional areas to age- and sex- matched dentate subjects

indicating the potential for maintaining a more satisfactory level of masticatory efficiency.

It has been proposed that the underlying defect in the neuromuscular system during ageing is a progressive motor neurone dysfunction and is first manifest by an increasing inability of the motor neurone to maintain its colony of muscle fibres in a fully viable condition.

When reviewing muscle function with age, consideration must also be given to the nervous system, as they are intimately related. It is well known that nerve cell loss is universal in old age and can be considered a true age-related change. Research has also indicated age-related changes in neurotransmitters, implying potential functional impairment in the elderly but further work is required. Peripheral nerve function usually declines with advancing age with a decrease in conduction velocity, increased latencies in multisynaptic pathways, decreased conduction at neuromuscular junctions and loss of receptors.

It has been proposed by some researchers that neurones may exert a trophic influence on such diverse tissues as skin, connective tissue and bone to the extent that withdrawal of its influence may determine the asset and speed of the ageing process throughout much of the remainder of the body.

Bone

Adult peak bone mass is attained at about 35 years. Subsequently, bone mass declines with age, with both cortical and trabecular bone being lost. There is an imbalance between resorption and replacement of bone in the Haversian systems. New Haversian systems are not completed so that the central canals

remain permanently wider than normal. One result of continuing subperiosteal osteoclastic activity in old age is the gradual increase in the diameter of some bones, with those of the skull similarly affected. This may account, in part, for the changes in facial appearance which often take place in advancing years.

Mandibular bone undergoes similar osteoporotic age changes to that found in other parts of the skeleton (**65, 66**), with mandibular bone density decreasing by around 20% between the ages of 45 and 90, women having significantly lower values throughout this age range. In addition to being less dense the bone is often more brittle and with increasing numbers of micro-fractures of the thinned trabeculae, healing occurs slowly owing to impaired remodelling. Also there is an increase in bone porosity, this being mainly due to an increase in vascular spaces.

At the cellular level, osteoblasts, which are derived from bone-lining cells, are severely depleted in number and activity by ageing and thus failure of osteoblastic production and function to keep pace with resorption is thought to be a key factor in long-term changes in skeletal form. This imbalance between osteoclastic and osteoblastic activity is exacerbated by the withdrawal of oestrogen during menopause. In addition, the elderly also have an impaired ability to increase calcium absorption in response to a low calcium diet; with the blood supply to older bones reduced, the supply and distribution of calcium salts will be affected. Changes to particular bony structures in the oral cavity may be affected or even accelerated by other factors. Although alveolar bone participates in the general loss of bone mineral with age by resorption of the bond matrix, this process may be accelerated by tooth loss, periodontal disease and inadequate or inappropriate prostheses in genetically susceptible individuals (**67**) or those with systemic disease.

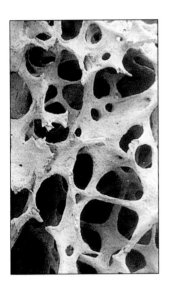

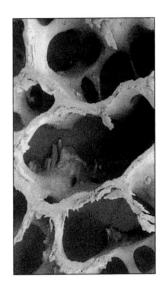

65 Section of sternum showing normal trabecular bone (far left) using SEM in a young male patient.

66 Section of sternum showing normal osteoporotic trabecular bone (near left) using SEM in an old male patient.

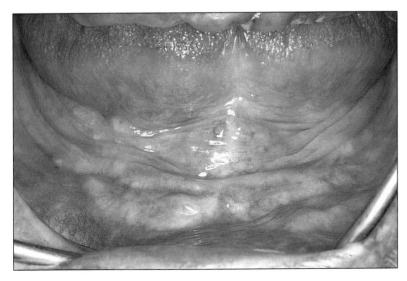

67 A very poor lower edentulous ridge in an elderly individual.

Temporomandibular joint

The situation with regard to the temporomandibular joint is unclear. A number of abnormalities including arthritic changes and deterioration of the meniscus have been reported but the relationship to and relative importance of age as distinct from local trauma and systemic disease is uncertain.

Conclusion

A more detailed knowledge of the normal ageing process would be beneficial in maintaining adequate oral function in the ageing patient and also in the diagnosis of disease, with possible improvement of their treatment through increased knowledge of the normal range.

Further reading

Ferguson, D.B. (ed.). 1987. *Frontiers of Oral Physiology – The Ageing Mouth*.

de Groot, J. & Chusid, J.G. *Ageing, Degeneration and Regeneration in Correlative Neuroanatomy*. Prentice-Hall, London.

Kenny, R.A. 1989. *Physiology of Aging – A Synopsis*. Year Book Medical Publishers Inc., London.

Papas, A.S., Niessen, L.C. & Chauncey, H.H. (eds). 1991. *Geriatric Dentistry – Aging and Oral Health*. Mosby–Year Book Inc., USA.

Yemm, R., Newton, J.P. & Lewis, G.R. 1986. Age changes in human muscle performance. In *Current Topics in Oral Biology*, eds S.J.W. Lisney & B. Matthews, pp. 17–25.

Woolf, A.D. & Dixon, A.St.J. 1988. *Osteoporosis – A Clinical Guide*. Martin Dintz, London.

5. The Dental Health of the Elderly Population

The dental health of an individual in any community relates to the fabric of the society in which the individual resides. External factors affect the dental state of today's elderly: education, income, mobility, availability of dentists, dental awareness and expectations, knowledge of the services provided and awareness of the possibilities and importance of dentistry.

In fairly recent times mass extractions were performed on young people, consequently many elderly people consider dentistry to be unpleasant, painful and costly (**68**). In the North of England and other parts of the United Kingdom, girls customarily had all teeth extracted and dentures constructed prior to marriage as part of their trousseau!

Slowly the public became aware of the advantages of dental treatment. In 1948, for example, in the United Kingdom the introduction of the National Health Service saw large numbers of people take the opportunity to remedy years of neglect. This sudden demand for treatment overwhelmed the profession and has led to high levels of edentulousness now found in the older United Kingdom population. Even now levels of edentulousness will remain high owing to the increase in size of the elderly population.

When contemplating surveys of the elderly it is important to consider the group or subgroup being examined; differences between social groups and sexes have already been highlighted. Surveys have been undertaken on many levels: some investigate treatment requirements, as assessed by the subjects themselves (perceived/subjective need) using postal questionnaires or interviews. Others attempt to assess amount and type of treatment needed by subject examination allowing comparison of normative and subjective need. Where subjects are examined, surveys are time-consuming and may neglect to consider that many subjects would fail to seek treatment and may refuse, were it to be offered. Care must be exercised when comparing results, as investigations undertaken in hospitals or long-stay institutions highlight problems of the infirm or psychogeriatric and often produce higher levels of need than results from surveys of elderly living in the community. Elderly people living at home tend to be fitter, more mobile and less handicapped. Since the dental state of today's elderly is related to the history of dental provision and attitudes over the whole life span of the individual and, since these factors vary greatly from one country to another, consideration of the dental state of the elderly worldwide will be on a national basis.

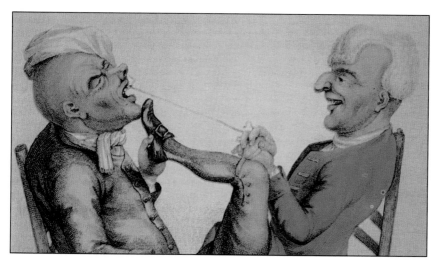

68 'An exercise in tooth-pulling'. Tom Bobbin (1810) *The Passions Humorously Delineated.* London.

United Kingdom – The early surveys

One of the first comprehensive surveys of the elderly was undertaken by Hobson and Roseman in 1949–50 when effects of the National Health Service (N.H.S.), which had by then provided free treatment for 2½ years, could be expected to be evident. Their survey, of elderly people living at home, showed that only 3.5% of men examined and 0.5% of women had adequate natural dentitions and that 41% of dentures were inadequate.

Comparison of this work with earlier studies – Humphrey (1889) and Sheldon (1948), just prior to implementation of the 1946 National Health Service (N.H.S.) Act – shows that, although population samples and examination methods were not matched, the proportion of older people using dentures increased over the 50 years (**Table 17**) and also greater use of dentures by women had

occurred. In addition to the fact that in 1948 dental treatment was free, factors causing these dramatic changes may have included, on a general level, improved education and health and, locally, factors affecting oral health and hygiene: increasing public awareness of dentistry, pollution, soft water, high atmospheric acid levels and mouth breathing. The survey by Hobson and Roseman formed an important baseline for later surveys: not only did they investigate edentulousness and denture adequacy but also examined public understanding about the way the N.H.S. worked and the influence of the cost of treatment. Attitudes to treatment were found to be class related: 10% of social class 1 and 2 (as defined by the British Registrar General) knew they needed treatment but made no attempt to obtain it; in Classes 4 and 5 the figure was 28.5%.

Table 17. Comparison of three early United Kingdom surveys.

Year	1889	1948	1953
Percentage of edentulous population not wearing dentures			
Women	51	7.7	3
Men	31	14.4	12
Percentage of sample wearing dentures			
Women	15.5	67	87
Men	14.0	40	62

United Kingdom Surveys, 1960 onwards

Several surveys undertaken in the late 1960s and early 1970s showed that the trend for high levels of edentulousness and widespread use of dentures continued (**Table 18**). These surveys of the general population highlighted problems of the elderly by comparison with younger people: Swallow and Adams examined a South Wales population and Bates and Murphy used the same group sampling only the edentulous among them. Bulman, Slack, Richards and Willcocks attempted to compare towns in the North and South of the country investigating both dental health and attitudes to dental health care and in 1968, the first Adult Dental Health Survey of England and Wales was undertaken followed in 1972 by the Scottish Dental Health Survey. Repetition of the Adult Dental Health Surveys every 10 years has provided fascinating and valuable data, showing regional variations in tooth

loss (**Table 19**), denture wearing and attitudes to dental treatment. Levels of edentulousness between 1968 and 1978 reduced nationally although, in 65–75-year-olds levels increased in the North. In the future, if these trends continue there should be more dentate individuals in the elderly group.

Analysing two communities, Bulman *et al.* compared Salisbury in Southern England, with fewer than the national average of dentists in relation to its population, to Darlington in northern England, which had more than the average number of dentists. In both areas levels of edentulousness were high: manual workers had lost more teeth than non-manual workers and 75% of people with retained teeth were assessed as needing treatment. This survey was one of the first to highlight differences between assessed and subjective need (**Table 20**). Two indicators of dental state are levels of

Table 18. Dental surveys of United Kingdom population including data on the elderly.

Survey	Year	Place	Sample	Age (Years)	Level of Edentulous (%)
Swallow and Adams	1967	SouthWales	745	15–74	45
				45	50
				55–64	80
				65+	100
Bulman, Slack, Richards and Willcocks	1965	Salisbury	65	61–70	87.5
			57	70+	90.6
	1968	Dalington	67	61–70	81.3
			55	70+	93.7
Adult Dental Health	1968	England and Wales	449	65–74	79
			338	75+	88
Adult Dental Health	1978		821	65–74	74
				75+	87
Adult Dental Health	1988		822	65–74	56
				75+	80
Scottish Dental Health	1972	Scotland	360	65–74	86
				75+	89
Scottish Dental Health	1978		227	65+	85
Scottish Dental Health	1988			65–74	63
				75+	84

Table 19. Regional variations in tooth loss (after Adult Dental Health Surveys): proportions (%) of people with no natural teeth.

Age (years)	The North			London and South East			England and Wales		
	1968	1978	1988	1968	1978	1988*	1968	1978	1988
45–54	55	32	22	27	21	8	41	29	15
55–64	73	62	53	55	31	22	64	48	36
65–74	81	87	74	69	60	44	79	74	56
75+	93	93	90	84	83	74	88	87	80

* Southern England

Table 20. Difference between perceived and assessed need in edentulous populations.

Survey	Perceived need (%)		Assessed need (%)
Bates and Murphy: South Wales 1968	Overall	17	No examination
	Male	14	
	Female	20	
Bulman, Slack, Richards and Willcocks:			
Salisbury 1965		12	64
Darlington 1965		12	40

Table 21. Levels of peridontal disease (%) in dentate adults over 35 years (after Adult Dental Health Survey 1988).

Age (years)	Some calculus	Deep pockets	Bleeding
35–44	93	13	81
45–54	96	17	81
55–64	96	16	77
>65	93	16	74

Table 22. Number of teeth extracted immediately prior to complete denture provision in people who had not previously worn a partial denture (after Adult Dental Health Surveys 1968 and 1978).

Number of teeth extracted	Became edentulous (%)	
	1948–1968	1968–1978
1–11	12	25
12–20	34	37
>21	54	38

periodontal disease (**Table 21**) and numbers of teeth extracted immediately prior to construction of complete upper and lower dentures (**Table 22**). The Adult Health Surveys show 96% of people over 55 had some form of periodontal problem. Many elderly people who might previously have had mass extractions are now likely to age with periodontally involved teeth requiring treatment and denture provision later in life. Increased tooth retention will lead to changed dental needs, with emphasis moving from complete denture provision to partial dentures, restorative and periodontal care needs. **Table 22** indicates altering treatment patterns: fewer large-scale clearances and increasing numbers experiencing partial dentures prior to becoming edentulous.

Later surveys of United Kingdom elderly focused on particular groups: elderly in institutional care were examined by Manderson and Ettinger, by Lemasney and Murphy and by Gerrish *et al.* Davidson assessed army pensioners (**Table 23**). Examination of people resident in the community was undertaken by Hamilton and by Smith and Sheiham who examined subjects attending two medical practices and by Diu and Gelbier who examined subjects attending a Community Care Centre. Taylor *et al.* examined 153 elderly people living at home and compared physically handicapped with non-handicapped subjects. Patients attending University College Hospital Dental School and inpatients in a geriatric hospital were surveyed by Ritchie; Whittle *et al.* examined elderly mentally ill in Salford. Some workers undertook interview or postal surveys. These surveys assessed demand for treatment and attitudes to dentistry but made no assessment of normative need. However, Hoad-Reddick (1991), following Palmer's lead, showed that care workers could assess need and produce a level close to normative need purely by questioning those in their care.

Similar findings emerged from these surveys: high levels of edentulousness, a lag between perceived and assessed need and, where subjects were examined, inadequate and dirty dentures and high levels of oral pathology. There are difficulties in making direct comparisons between different residential groups: people in residential accommodation may receive assistance with dental hygiene but find access to care by a dentist difficult if the home owner does not understand the need for regular dental care of the elderly (**Table 24**)

In an attempt to compare groups directly, Hoad-Reddick interviewed and examined 1% of the Halton Health Authority (Cheshire) selected with comparable residential groups representative of the overall community. Differences in perceived need were found to be highly significant between groups and were also age related. Overall normative need was 84.95%, with subjects in institutionalised care being more likely to need treatment than those caring for themselves in the community (**Table 25**). Of particular concern is the high level of oral pathology discovered in many surveys (**Table 26**).

Table 23. Later United Kingdom Surveys.

Survey	Year	Place	Number	Exam/Postal	Level of edentulousness(%)	Perceived need (%)	Normative Need(%)
Institutional Residents							
Gerrish, Yardley *et al.*	1971	Cardiff	327	Exam	86.9	34	46
Manderson and Ettinger	1975	Edinburgh	442	Exam	90.7	39	70.5
Lemasney and Murphy	1984	Ireland	368	Exam	78	27	63
Army Pensioners							
Davidson	1979	Royal Hospital Chelsea	375	Exam	75.7	25	70.3
Community/Medical Practice							
Smith and Sheiham	1980	Nottingham	254	Exam	74	42	78
Hamilton	1985	Salford	210	Exam	70	35	85 Pros.
Taylor King and Sheiham	1986	Grimsby	153	Exam	83	29	50
Diu and Gelbier	1989	Lambeth Com. Centre	293	Exam	63.5	53	82
Hospital in-patients							
Ritchie	1973	U.C.H. London	300	Exam	70.6	50	92
Whittle	1987	Salford (mentally ill)	117*	Exam	92	16	68
					87	19	70
General							
Hoad-Reddick	1985	Halton H.A. Cheshire	233	Exam	88	25.3	84.9
Postal/Interview surveys							
Palmer	1977	Somerset	404	Interview	83	18	–
Osborne, Maddick, Gould and Ward	1979	Hampshire	2460	Postal	–	22	–
Kail and Silver	1984	Herts.	294	Interview	84.6	33	–
Broadway and Kemp	1985	East Anglia	2000	Interview			

* 57 ill, 60 control

Table 24. Factors causing differences between surveys.

1.	Age Group
2.	Sex
3.	Ethnic origin
4.	Residential status
5.	Education
6.	Regional differences
7.	Financial status – cost of treatment
8.	Social status/class
9.	Rural versus urban dwellers

Table 25. Comparison of different residential groups (Hoad–Reddick).

	Longstay (LSH) hospitals (%)	Elderly peoples homes (EPH) (%)	Community with assistance (CWA) (%)	No assistance in the Community (NAC) (%)	Total
Number of subjects	55	62	63	53	233
Perceived need	9.3	24.2	27.0	37.7	25.3
Concern over dentures	71.4	76.5	70.6	75	73.8
Concern over retained teeth	28.6	23.6	31.4	25.0	26.2
Attendance pain	95	95.1	96.7	89.8	94.3
Regular	5	4.9	3.3	10.2	5.7
Assessed need	88.4	70.7	70.9	68.0	85
Lag between perceived and assessed need	79.1	46.5	43.9	30.3	59.7
Dirty dentures	45.5	73.8	52.5	61.9	60.3
Named dentures	33.3	6.4	8.0	2.3	10.5
Pathology	14	31	38.7	68	38.3
Number of lost dentures	12	9	3	1	25

Table 26. Levels of oral pathology – comparison of different surveys.

Survey	Year	Percentage of subjects with oral pathology	Place of residence
Ritchie	1973	49	Dental Hospital/Geriatric ward
Manderson and Ettinger	1975	50	Institutionalised
Smith and Sheiham	1980	60	At home in the community
Hoad-Reddick	1985	38	14 LSH
			31 EPH
			38 NAC
			68 CWA
Diu and Gelbier	1989	48	Community assisted
Hamilton	1990	49	Community
			55 denture wearers
			16 non-denture wearers

LSH, long-stay hospital.
EPH, elderly people's homes.
NAC, no assistance in the community.
CWA, community with assistance.

In the Hamilton sample oral pathology was found in 14% of those in long-stay hospitals and 68% of those caring for themselves in the community. Those in the community, although more aware of need for treatment, are more likely to suffer oral pathology owing to a lack of regular contact with dentists or nurses. High levels of assessed need in hospitals may be partly accounted for by lost dentures or non-replacement of very old dentures, whereas in old people's homes, or elderly in the community with no assistance, it may be due to lack of contact with dentists and lack of understanding of, or interest in, dental problems by caring staff. Other problems highlighted were large numbers of dirty dentures in old people's homes (73.8%) and a higher proportion of lost dentures in long-stay hospitals. Clearly, there should be a drive to educate denture wearers and carers of the importance of, and means of achieving, adequate denture cleansing. The need for naming all dentures upon manufacture is demonstrated.

Deterrents to visiting a dentist

Having established the nature of the problem of poor dental health in the elderly, interest focused on reasons for non-attendance at a dentist or reluctance to accept treatment when it was offered (**Table 27**). Causes of non-attendance tend to be multifactorial: failing health in the individual, cost of treatment, lack of understanding of dentistry or fear related to poor experiences when younger.

Table 27. Factors affecting attendance.

Mobility
Poor general health
Transport problems
Fear
Lack of understanding of dental care
Cost
Poor knowledge of services provided

The Wider World

In many developed countries interest in geriatric dentistry has been pursued with similar or even greater vigour to that in the United Kingdom. Worldwide there is a similarity between results of surveys and factors affecting demand. Initial high levels of edentulousness are unique to the United Kingdom and related to historical attitudes of dentistry and the subsidised service provided by the N.H.S. It is pleasing to observe levels of edentulous elderly seem set to reduce. In less-fortunate, less-developed areas of the world, dentistry is not advanced and dentist: population ratios are low. Prospects of improvement in the field of geriatric dentistry seem bleak: proportions of dentate elderly are high, although their dental state is poor. In less-advanced countries life expectancy is still low, as the great increase in numbers of elderly people has not occurred: other health problems are considered of greater importance than the state of their mouths and teeth.

The United States

North American social attitudes to tooth loss differed from those in the United Kingdom. Most dental care is undertaken in private practice: one-third of the population has some form of dental insurance. People over 65 are helped by the Federal Government's Medicare plan covering oral surgical services. The United States Department of Health has monitored tooth loss nationwide. Since levels of

Table 28. Comparison of tooth loss in United States of America with England and Wales (after 1968 Adult Health Survey).

Age (Years)	United Kingdom		United States of America	
	Male	Female	Male	Female
45–54	36.1	44.2	20.0	20.1
55–64	61.1	66.1	34.7	38.0
65–74	77.6	79.6	45.1	53.0
75+	87.7	88.3		
75–79	–	–	55.7	65.6

edentulousness in the United States are lower than in the United Kingdom, the same degree of reduction cannot be anticipated **(Table 28)**. In such a large, varied and multiracial country there is considerable regional variation of education, residential status, social status, wealth, etc.

Taylor and Doku assessed the oral conditions of a cross-section of all elderly, as they felt earlier surveys of institutionalised elderly were complicated by 'disease, regimented diets and inadequate oral hygiene' and only accounted for 5% of the elderly. Their elderly sample attended the Age Centre of New England and excluded anyone with impaired health. The 29% level of edentulous is low compared with other surveys **(Table 29)** but there was considerable unmet normative need: only one-third of dentures were satisfactory, 93% of dentate women had gingival recession and 71% of male and 59% of female denture wearers were satisfied with their dentures. Temporomandibular joint problems (clicking) affected over 50% of their sample, although only 22.1% of dentate and 10% of edentulous individuals felt pain. By 69 years of age the majority had retained just over one-half of their teeth. Thereafter tooth loss accounted for approximately one tooth per year.

Ettinger and Beck using the National Centre of Health's statistics showed that in 1976 more than 50% of all over 65 years were edentulous and, although in 1978 56% of the total United States population visited a dentist, only 35% of the over 60s had sought treatment. There may have been a small improvement in the previous decade since, in 1971, 72% of elderly had not visited a dentist in the previous 5 years and in geriatric institutions 6.2% had no dentures, 8.9% never wore them, 4.6% wore them only infrequently and one-quarter of those with dentures thought they needed treatment. There is considerable perceived need, although subjects may not seek treatment.

Almost 50% of over 65-year-olds in America have some teeth: many papers discuss problems of restorative care in this group. The incidence of coronal and root caries followed over 3 years showed a greater annual growth rate of root carious lesions per 100 susceptible surfaces than of coronal caries. In Alabama, Wallace *et al.* examined 608 subjects and found that 69.7% had at least two root carious lesions, with the highest incidence in lower second premolars. Significantly higher levels of root caries occurred in white than in black subjects and more in men than in women **(Table 30)**. Hand *et al.* found, over 3 years, that 2% of previously dentate became edentulous – women retained teeth in one arch whereas men became totally edentulous. He was unable to predict which subjects were most at

Table 29. Comparison of edentulism in North American Surveys 1963–88.

Survey	Year	Place	Age	Edentulous (%)	Normative need (%)
Taylor and Doku	1963	New England healthy	52–92	29	edentulous, 69.5; dentate (periodontal) problems, 88.2
Ettinger and Beck	1980	Iowa	65–74	33.8	
			75+	44.4	
Ettinger, Beck and Jakobsen	1986	National Centre for Health Statistics	65+	50	
Simpson *et al.*	1983	Nursing home Residents	65+	50	
Hand *et al.*	1988	Iowa (rural)	65+	37.8	Dentate 81

Table 30. Sexual and racial differences in root caries incidence (after Wallace, Birmingham, Alabama).

	%
Black	57.7
White	77.9
Male	76.1
Female	65.5

risk of becoming totally edentulous owing to the large numbers of variables.

Ettinger *et al.* (1988) analysed examinations of 853 nursing home residents. Using medical charts without dental examinations they projected who needed dental care but not who would accept treatment. Lack of dentures was the major factor affecting need for treatment.

Despite the decline in edentulism, the need for treatment will remain high into the next century. Demand will increase for partial dentures and, owing to improved education and increased awareness, treatment uptake will increase. Johansen *et al.* may be showing the way forward with their research into the remineralisation of root and coronal lesions using an experimental regime on 171 subjects: root caries remineralised to a greater extent.

Clearly, there is a need for greater oral health instruction to accompany changes in the ageing dentition. Younger elderly tend to be better educated than older elderly and may be more receptive to educational programmes.

Canada

The dentist : population ratio (1:1925) is similar to that in the United States (**Table 31**). No countrywide subsidised service exists, although government assistance is available for the 'needy'. Less than one-third of the population have dental insurance. Canadian over 65s were investigated by a number of studies. **Table 32** suggests some reduction in overall numbers of edentulous although survey populations are not matched. MacEntee *et al.* found high levels of normative need but felt that less than 10% of denture wearers would have benefited from treatment, whereas 60% of dentate required restorations and 35% needed extractions. Mandibular dysfunction occurred in

Table 31. Dentist : population ratios in the United Kingdom, United States of America, Canada, Australia, New Zealand and Japan.

Country	Dentist : population ratio
Japan	1 : 1767
United States of America	1 : 1784
Canada	1 : 1925
Australia	1 : 2375
United Kingdom	1 : 2569
New Zealand	1 : 2682

Table 32. Varying levels of edentulousness in Canadian surveys 1969–85.

Survey	Sample size	Type	Year	Age (years)	Edentulous (%)		Normative need (%)
Lightman, (Toronto)	491	Nursing home	1969	60+	81		
Martinello and Leake, (Ontario)	517	Nursing home	1971	60+	77		
Kandelman and Lepage, (Quebec)	956	Cross-section of Canada	1982	65+	72 at home nursing home hospital	71.4 80 74.6	75.4
MacEntee *et al.*	250	Long-term institution	1985	60+	70		>50

25%, oral mucosal pathology was rare although 20% displayed one inflammatory, hyperkeratotic or atrophic disorder of the mucosa (the incidence was higher in 24-h denture wearers). The 1978–79 Canadian Health Survey showed that 67% of elderly had not visited a dentist in the previous 5 years (a lower figure than in the United States) (**Table 33**). However, one must take into account the large number of denturists compared with other countries (**Table 34**). Barriers of demand are similar to those in the United Kingdom.

Table 33. Percentage of subjects over 65 who had not visited a dentist in the last one and five years.

Country		Last year (%)	Last five years (%)
Canada		77	67
United States of America (non-institutionalised)		42.6	40
United Kingdom (age 55+)	1968	27	
	1978	32 (dentate)	

1978–79, Canadian Health Survey.
1981, US National Health Interview Survey.
1978, Adult Health Survey.

Table 34. Ratio of dentists to denturists in four countries with similar dentist : population ratios (after FDI).

Country	Dentist : population	Dentist : denturist	No. denturist
United States of America	1 : 1784	700 : 1	197
Canada	1 : 1925	5.05 : 1	2700
Australia	1 : 2375	11.4 : 1	607
United Kingdom	1 : 2569		0

Australia

Surveys in this country are difficult to compare directly because of the geographical isolation of parts of the population. Private health insurance covers 42.5% of people and some subsidised clinics provide care to Aborigines. A postal survey in Victoria was conducted separately to assess dental need: 51.9% of his elderly sample's dentures were over 10 years old, suggesting few review or follow-up appointments. Lack of motivation and finance were the main barriers to treatment. Levels of edentulousness may be reducing (**Table 35**). Women were more likely to be edentulous than men but other factors such as urban versus rural dwellers, dentist:patient ratios, or geographic isolation affected samples. In Bussleton, Western Australia 4% of the edentulous had no dentures; in South Australia the level was 15%. **Table 34** shows the high level of denturists in Australia, which may affect attendances at dental surgeries.

Table 35. Reduction in edentulousness in Australia 1970–78.

Survey	Year	Place	Age (years)	Edentulousness %
Evans and Cellier	1970	South Australia	70+	90
Roder and Selge	1974	South Australia	65+	
				78.9 (male)
				93.5 (female)
Medcalf	1976	Western Australia	70+	81
Spratley	1978	Victoria	65+	68.5

New Zealand

Surveys undertaken between 1950 and 1976 demonstrate over 80% edentulousness in the over 60s (**Table 36**). Future trends look promising, with less tooth loss in the 35–44 age group. Total edentulousness was related to social class (0% Class I : 64% Class V), 60% of denture wearers required treatment and 62.3% wore a denture more than 10 years old. Women had better oral health than men and in 1968 more had retained 19 teeth – considered the minimum necessary by the FDI. Fluoride was added to drinking water first in 1954 and by 1984 should have reached half the population. Thus, although dental health in New Zealand seems set to improve, the elderly will still present with problems, especially as dentistry is private practice based with some social welfare or Hospital Dentistry for means-tested people.

Table 36. Edentulousness in New Zealand 1950–84.

Survey	Year	Edentulous % age 60+	Edentulous % age 35–44
Davis and Walsh	1950	80	42
Burgess and Black	1968	84	64
Robertson	1976	82	28
Ross	1984		16

The Indian Sub-Continent

Dental provision that is very different from the developed world is illustrated in **69, 70**. But, in a country where the dentist : population ratio is 1:200 985, treatment relates mainly to pain relief and oral surgery. Normally, treatment is on a fee for service basis, although public dental services are available in primary health centres, government dispensaries in villages and in dental hospitals. A survey of geriatric patients attending a dental college and hospital in Calcutta found demand low due to two factors: low awareness of oral health, and habitation remote from dental clinics. Files of 60 900

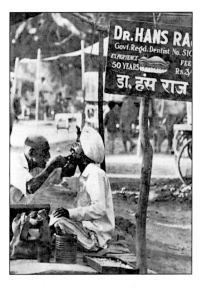

69 Indian subcontinent: dentistry performed in the open air.

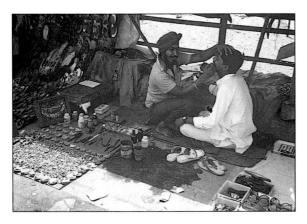

70 Dentures for sale in a street market (Indian sub-continent).

patients collected over 20 years (**Table 37**) showed that the majority required tooth extraction and denture provision. Use of preventive measures and oral health awareness were virtually non-existent.

In other countries of the Indian sub-Continent even less is known about the dental health of the elderly.

Table 37. Treatment provided to 60 000 geriatric patients 1967–86 Calcutta.

Department	%
Department of Oral and Maxillo-Facial Surgery	71
Periodontology	5.70
Conservative Dentistry	3.62
Oral Pathology and Bacteriology	3.73
Prosthodontics (partial dentures: 607	
Complete dentures 9891)	17.24

The Far East

In many countries of this region traditional dentistry exists alongside new advanced techniques: many practising dentists have received no formal training.

China

In the 1950s, Mao encouraged population increase. The resultant population bulge of 30–40-year-olds has stimulated research into ageing and problems of the elderly. The Beijing Institute of Gerodontology investigated 2190 people over 60 years: 12.6% were edentulous and 9.5% had intact dentitions. Of those over 80, 71% had some retained teeth (average 13.5) compared with only 20% in the United Kingdom. However, tooth retention is not without problems; 92% of dentate showed evidence of decay, 98% showed wear with 70–80% being advanced into the dentine. Where dental awareness is low and provision scarce, tooth loss and advanced periodontal destruction are not inevitable (**71**). Mean attachment loss was only 5 mm, which may account for the low incidence of root surface caries average number of lesions, 1.8 active and 1.5 passive. Cervical abrasion was age related and greatest in the upper jaw, possibly caused by incorrect tooth cleaning (**72**). Walls, visiting China noted

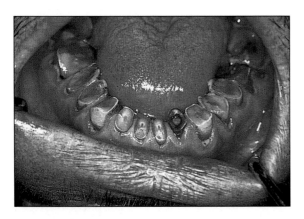

71 China: advanced tooth surface loss without advanced periodontal disease. Owing to the scarcity of dental care many broken down teeth are retained.

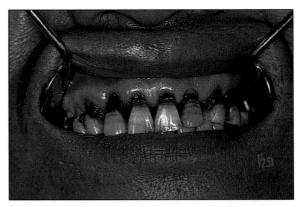

72 China: cervical abrasion and decay. Poor tooth cleaning and lack of dental care lead to high levels of unmet need.

widespread incorrect use of toothpicks and brushes. He also felt unmet need was large: 15% of edentulous and 68% of partly edentate were without dentures. He stated 'it is unlikely that need can be satisfied in the foreseeable future due to low numbers of dental personnel available'.

Japan

Japan has the fastest-ageing society in the world, yet a postal survey of dental schools shows no school teaching geriatric dentistry as a specialty and 17.5% do not teach it at all. In 1986, the Japanese Association for Geriatric Dentistry was founded as 'the status of Japanese geriatric dentistry is still in its infancy compared to the USA'. Takagi *et al.* surveyed tooth life expectancy and found higher numbers of retained teeth in women, although edentulousness was also high (**Table 38**).

Table 38. Comparison of DMF rates of elderly in the Far East with the United Kingdom (unmatched groups).

Country	Year	Age (years)	DMF	With teeth (%)	Mean no. teeth
Philippines	1984	65+	20.3		
Malaysia	1984	65+	25		
Japan	1958	80+	25		
China	1989	80+		71	13.5
United Kingdom	1988	65-74		44	
		75+		20	

Malaysia

New subjects attending the University Dental Faculty in Kuala Lumpur showed greatest demand for dentures (36%), extractions (21.6%) and treatment of toothache (15.5%), although examination found greatest need for extractions (55.3%). Much need was unrecognised by subjects – one-third did not perceive caries or periodontal disease as problems. These results, although probably atypical of the whole country because of the larger proportions of women attending and the sample being from an urban population, may indicate the trend. Razak and Alis report that remarkably little is known of the dental status of the elderly in this country.

Ignorance of dental health and dentistry, lack of money and fear of conservative treatment meant that up to 54.7% of the adult population needed some sort of denture. The picture for the elderly is bleak – high DMF rates (**Table 38**), high levels of edentulousness and scant denture provision. However, improvements are likely owing to the expansion of dental services, extensive health education and introduction of fluoride programmes.

Europe, Scandinavia and beyond

Surveys in Europe have mainly been confined to the northern part of the Continent. It is expected that with development of the Free European Market from 1992 and increasing exchange visits between dental professions, research into gerodontology will spread to the more southern countries. As elsewhere in the world, direct comparison of surveys is unreliable owing to many variables. Europe is a very wide and varying continent – comparison of isolated fishing/farming communities with city dwellers or northern mountainous regions with southern mediterranean climes is obviously difficult. However, comparisons do indicate trends and, as in other developed countries it will be shown that edentulousness is decreasing. The dental profession is faced with an enlarging dentate elderly population and its attendant problems. The dentist:population ratio is generally similar, although Spain, Portugal and Turkey have considerably higher ratios.

Surveys spanning 10 years in Denmark and Sweden (**Table 39**) show at least 10% reduction in levels of edentulousness, even when sampling differences are taken into account.

As in the United Kingdom and the United States, rural dwellers show poorer dental states than urban dwellers, women tend to have higher levels of edentulousness than men and individuals in higher social classes are more regular attenders and have more teeth than those in lower social groups. Denture provision varies and is related to availability of dentists but also to ability to pay. In Ireland, two surveys of geriatric patients show only one-quarter of the edentulous wearing dentures (**Table 40**). The elderly are poor utilisers of dental services: in Denmark, only 15% were regular attenders, although dentate individuals were more likely to have visited the dentist recently than edentulous individuals (**Table 41**). Clearly, the need for continued dental care and regular examination must be widely publicised.

The incidence of oral pathology in many countries is worryingly high (**Table 42**) and in many surveys, levels greater than 50% have been discovered. Great differences between perceived and assessed need are demonstrated – unless the elderly are aware of problems they are unlikely to attend for treatment. Later surveys of dentate elderly highlighted problems of gingivitis and root caries. Some workers have used DMF rates to measure problems in the dentate; this seems an inappropriate index as no account is taken of the periodontal condition, yet it does indicate patterns of disease. In Scandinavia, DMF rates for women were higher than for men owing to an increased number of fillings and greater attendance at dental surgeries. Numbers of retained teeth has also been used as an index, but this takes no account of their state. In Denmark, Grabowski and Bertram found an average of 4.9 sound teeth in a dentate population with a mean number of 12 retained teeth. Vigild, investigating levels of periodontal disease, found it worse in the institutionalised and where staff were responsible for tooth cleaning. Wirz in Switzerland, found carers had received little instruction in oral health care.

Table 39. Surveys of Denmark and Sweden showing reducing edentulousness during the 1970s and 1980s.

Country/Survey	Year	Age (years)	Type	Edentulous (%)	Need (%) Assessed	Need (%) Perceived
Denmark						
Grabowski and Bertram	1975	65+	Cross-section	68.2	71.8	Edent. } 25
				64.7 F, 70.7 M	96.6	Dent. } 80
Christensen	1977	65–77	Cross-section	66		
Brauer *et al.*	1985	65+	Hospital	58	82 { 66 Pros.	25
					46 Cons/Perio	
					38 Oral Surg.	
Vigild	1987		Nursing home	74	67 19	} realistic
				80 F, 62 M		
			Hospital	62	71 32	
				71 F, 47 M		
Sweden						
Christrom	1970	60+	Nursing Home	75		25 Edent. no denture
Marken and Hedengaard	1970	60–84	Random	39		
Barenthin	1977	65+		70		24
Thorselius	1981	83.9 (mean)	Old Peoples Homes	66		3 Edent. no denture
Ostberg	1981	65–84		52.5		
				50 F, 55 M		
Hugoson and Koch	1982	60–70	Random	20		
		70+		37		
Palmquist	1986	65+	Rural population	38.5		

Table 40. Edentulousness in four European countries.

Country/Survey	Year	Type	Age (years)	Edentulous (%)			Need (%)		
				Total	Male	Female	Assessed		Perceived
Norway									
Rise and Heloe	1978	Cross-section	65–79	77	89	72		97	
Switzerland									
Stuck *et al.*	1989	Geriatric hospital	66–95	59.4			Dentate	97.8	30.4
							Edent.	31.5	13.1
Ireland									
Lemasney									
and Murphy	1983	Geriatric hospital	58–99	78	69	91			
Corridan	1965	General hospital. Chronic sick	elderly	74.5	66	80	Dentate	91	
							Overall	83.4	
Finland									
Vehkalahti									
and Paunio	1988	General population	65+		51	65			
Ekelund	1988	Old Peoples Homes	65+	68				96	
Tuominen *et al.*	1984	Cross-section population	65+	59.6					60–69 11.0
									70+ 12.6
Makila	1977	Nursing homes	65+	67	60	69			

Table 41. Health service usage by European elderly.

Country	Year of survey	Regular attenders (%)	
		Edentulous	Dentate
Finland	1987	10.1	30.3
Denmark	1975	11.7	48.9
Sweden (last attended	1982	50	
< 3 years)	1986	43 69	84
Norway (last attended	1978	17	
< 5 years)			
United Kingdom (last	1979	18	43
attended < 5 years)			

Table 42. Oral pathology in Northern Europe (see also **Table 26**).

Survey	Year	Country	Type	Subjects with oral pathology (%)
Ekelund	1988	Finland	Residential homes	60
Brauer *et al.*	1986	Norway	Geriatric hospital	52
Grabowski and Bertram	1975	Denmark	Denture wearers	64.8
Marken and Hedegard	1970	Sweden	Elderly in Stockholm	57
Thorselius	1981	Sweden	Old peoples home in Gothenburg	39
Hoad-Reddick	1989	United Kingdom	Cross-section of elderly	38

Israel

The dentist : population ratio (1:1010) is similar to that of many countries in Europe. For the majority, payment is made direct to the dentist, although many local authorities provide a school dental service and thus improvement in dental health can be expected in later generations. Israel is a multi-racial society. A survey of 260 elderly nursing-home residents found ethnic trends related to tooth loss and denture usage. Dentures were worn by 78% of edentulous American-Europeans but by only 56% Afro-Asians. Whereas no American-Europeans had naturally functioning dentitions, a significant number of Afro-Asians did. Differences in number of subjects with pathology also varied significantly between groups. Factors other than racial differences may account for variations – amount of education, place of residence, origin, presence or absence of dentures. High levels of retained teeth may indicate dental neglect rather than high levels of care; Mersel *et al.* found only 13.7% of dentures worn were satisfactory (**Table 43**).

Table 43. Edentulousness in Israeli Surveys 1975–89.

Survey	Year	Type	Age (years)	Edentulous/ no denture (%)		Normative need (%)
Langer *et al.*	1975	Institution	75+	62.3	Male	
				75.9	Female	
Mersel *et al.*	1984	Jerusalem retired	60+	54		86.3
Mann *et al.*	1985	Mixed	65+	59.5		87.5
Pisanty *et al.*	1989	Nursing Home	60+	34.4		

Surgery design for access by elderly patients

Major barriers to seeking treatment have been shown to be mobility, failing eyesight, cost and fear often based on lack of understanding of modern dentistry. **Table 44** shows major physical problems affecting elderly attending for treatment.

Access

Consideration should be given to site of the practice:
- Accessible for public transport.
- Providing good parking facilities.
- Easy entrance to the practice with ramps rather than steps.

Within the building

Where patients have problems with mobility or eyesight, they may need assistance or need space for walking aids/zimmers or wheelchairs. Space should be available:
- At doorways.
- In corridors.
- Within the surgery.
- At the side of the chair (**73**).

The waiting area

Many elderly people have impaired vision or may feel anxious about the appointment. Too many notices may confuse the patient: clear type should be used. Chairs in waiting rooms ideally should provide good back support and have arm rests. (**74**).

In the surgery

Chairs

Upright dental chairs are more acceptable to elderly people than flat couches (**75, 76**). Chairs should be sited to allow easy access, if arm rests are removable it is easier for the assistant to help the patient to be seated (**73, 75**).

74 This type of chair provides good support whilst seated. Arms provide assistance on rising.

Table 44. Major problems affecting elderly while visiting the dentist.

1.	Mobility:	inability to walk
		walking aids
		wheelchair
2.	Sight	
3.	Hearing	
4.	Medical problems	
5.	Postural instability (problems lying down and then getting up)	
6.	Fear (heart rate may increase)	
7.	Incontinence	

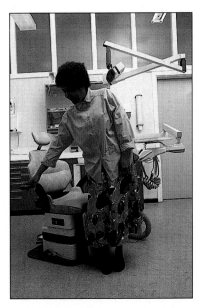

73 A dental chair providing clear access for an elderly person (note the removable arm rest).

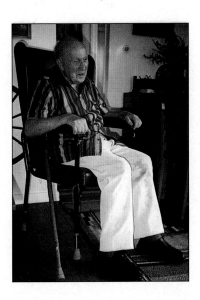

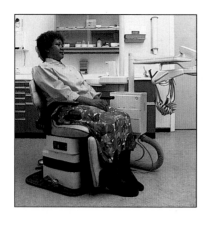

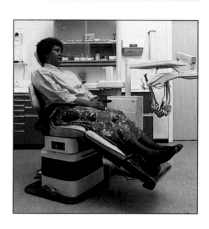

75 Dental chair which provides easy access owing to the absence of a step for feet and also allows patient to remain in a sitting position.

76 Same chair with legs supported.

Lighting

Failing eyesight often affects ability to adapt to changing light effects. Thus, pooling of light should be avoided – maintain even lighting throughout.

Outlining doors and doorways a different colour from surrounding walls makes movement around the practice easier.

Noise levels

As hearing deteriorates extrinsic noises can affect patients: background noises make speech detection difficult. Noisy pieces of equipment should be sited outside the surgery if possible (**Table 45**).

Table 45. Appliances that may produce unnecessary background noise — site outside the surgery if possible.

Heaters	Telephone
Compressor	Steriliser
Vacuum Motor	Saliva ejector
Amalgamator	Laboratory (if on the premises)

The appointments and desk/reception area

- Provide written instructions additional to verbal advice. (Memory deteriorates with age and when agitated elderly people may not take in instructions.)
- Use very clear writing, preferably printed.
- Avoid large numbers of notices/adverts: these will be very confusing to anxious or poorly sighted elderly people.
- Clear notices for toilet and exit. (Where elderly are incontinent they may be made especially anxious if not told where the nearest toilet is situated.)
- In order to keep anxiety threshold as low as possible, explain exact details of: treatment, waiting time, siting of surgery. Give elderly patients plenty of time. Often they meet very few people during the course of the day.
- Allow the nurse as far as possible to sit with them to reassure them before and after appointments if they are confused or anxious.

Further reading

Ettinger, R.L., Beck, J.D. & Jakobsen, J. 1988. Prediction of need and acceptance of dental services for institutionalised patients. *Gerodontics*, **4**, 109–13.

Hoad-Reddick, G. 1991. A study to determine oral health needs of institutionalised elderly patients by non-dental health workers. *Dentistry and Oral Epidemiology*, **19**(4), 233–6.

Kandelman, D., Bordeur, J.M. & Simard, P. 1986. Dental needs of the elderly: a comparison between some European and North American Surveys. *Community Dental Health*, **3**, 19–39.

Office of Population Censuses and Surveys. 1990. *Adult Dental Health 1988 United Kingdom*. HMSO, London.

6. Periodontal Care and Prevention

The nature of periodontal disease

Dental plaque, the accumulation of bacterial deposits on the tooth surface, represents part of the oral commensal bacterial flora. The response of the gingival marginal tissue to this bacterial deposit is manifest as gingivitis. Gingivitis, like the plaque itself, is virtually a universal finding in populations of all age groups and varies only in extent and severity. We have come to regard gingivitis as a disease process largely because it may progress to the more serious condition of periodontitis, which ultimately threatens tooth support and possibly the integrity of the entire dentition.

Thirty years of intensive research on a worldwide scale has conclusively demonstrated that the development and progression of periodontitis is dependent on the activity of dental plaque micro-organisms and particularly those in the subgingival area, possibly potentiated by the presence of subgingival calculus. The interaction between the micro-organisms and the host response is extremely complex and depends upon a systemically based activation of inflammatory and immune components. These, in turn, are largely governed in their activity by genetic mechanisms. The subgingival plaque flora is potentially comprised of over 300 bacterial species and others that remain to be identified and classified. The equally diverse host responses demonstrate elements of inflammation and immunity, both cellular and humoral. Of particular interest have been the studies demonstrating that some auto-immune type reactions may be significant in giving rise to tissue destruction. The genetic basis for individual responses in immunological, inflammatory and infective diseases has recently received considerable attention. It is now possible to apply some of these principles to studies of oral diseases, including periodontal diseases, and there is increasing evidence that genetic factors may be particularly important in conferring high susceptibility or high resistance to the progression of tissue destruction. The principles of interaction within this system are illustrated in **77**.

The concept of resistance and susceptibility in periodontal diseases is no different to that for other such disease processes. Moreover, many of the potentially destructive mechanisms have analogies with other biological activities, including the ageing process. For example, neutrophil granulocytes, the predominant defence cells within gingival crevicular fluid whether in health or disease, provide the initial and most important inflammatory defence in all mammalian species. While containing an impressive array of enzymes able to inhibit many bacterial mechanisms, their most important role is in producing oxygen radicals and ionic species that are highly toxic to bacteria over a wide spectrum. When the cell membrane is stimulated, molecular oxygen, taken in through the membrane, is rapidly reduced in a stepwise process, ultimately to water. The intermediate stages, however, produce the superoxide anion, hydrogen peroxide and, via the activity of the enzyme myeloperoxidase, hypochlorous acid (HOCl), an extremely potent

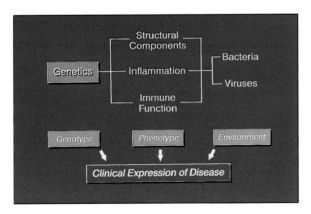

77 Schematic representation of interactions between genetically determined host factors and the microbial environment. Theoretically, a very large range of clinical outcomes are possible.

antibacterial agent. The essential steps of this reaction are shown in **78** and an important feature of this process is that a high proportion of the reaction products are released to the extracellular environment where they further potentiate the antibacterial function of these cells, although most killing occurs intracellularly. However, as well as being effective against the bacteria, the host tissues are also damaged. While this process defends the integrity of the organism as a whole, there is a price to be paid in the form of local tissue destruction. Oxidation effects may be directed towards structural proteins producing cross-linking and also towards DNA by contributing to the well-recognised biochemical manifestations of the ageing process. The production of 'detoxifying' enzymes such as superoxide dismutase (SOD) and catalase are largely under genetic control and their loci in many animal species, including humans, have been identified.

The hypothesis is that these processes including many others in the inflammatory and immunological responses, are variably active within different individuals or even between different populations. Equally, the pathogenic potential of dental plaque bacteria is now regarded as variable, and specific not only to individuals but to certain sites within the mouth. It is possible that periodontal disease progresses in random bursts of activity rather than as a continuum once started. Although still not universally accepted, there is much support for this theory and many clinicians would confirm that this explains the manifestations of disease as seen in their own patients. The scheme is further complicated by the additional influence of systemic factors such as hormonal disturbances, iron deficiency, both psychological and physical stress and many other disease processes. Early-onset forms of periodontitis have been recognised for many years but particularly investigated over the past two decades. For example, both local and generalised forms of juvenile periodontitis, prepubertal periodontitis and adult rapidly progressive periodontitis have been shown to develop in the presence of particularly aggressive subgingival bacteria, but equally have a susceptibility component related to inflammatory and immune dysfunction. The concept that gingivitis inevitably leads to tooth loss through periodontitis in middle and later years has now been effectively challenged and indeed refuted through widespread epidemiological investigations. Until the results of such studies became available, there have been instances when finding an elderly patient with healthy periodontal support was thought worthy of special comment.

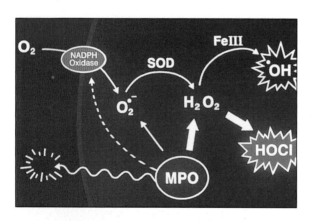

78 The oxygen-dependent microbiocidal system of neutrophil granulocytes, of which approximately 1×10^{11} are produced by the bone marrow daily. The membrane-bound NADPH oxidase enzyme reduces oxygen to water via several crucial stages. Powerful radicals such as superoxide anion (O_2^-), hydrogen peroxide (H_2O_2) and the hydroxyl radical (OH) may kill bacteria, but also damage host tissues. Myeloperoxidase (MPO) potentiates the protective effects by converting much of the H_2O_2 to hypochlorous acid (HOCL) and other enzymes help to regulate the process (e.g. superoxide dismutase, SOD)

Epidemiology of periodontal diseases and the ageing population

The now encyclopaedic information obtained from the many laboratory and clinically based studies on the aetiology and pathogenesis of periodontal disease has been complemented by large-scale epidemiological investigations conducted in virtually all geographical regions of the world. Data from undeveloped, developing and post-industrialised nations all support the concept of the spectrum of resistance and susceptibility within adult populations. This includes studies carried out in countries in which there is no organised dental care. The vast majority of such surveys are cross-sectional in nature and generally provide data from all age groups. The overall conclusion is that only a small proportion of any adult population is susceptible to advanced destructive disease leading to substantial tooth loss at an early age. An equally small proportion, generally 3–10%, appears to be highly resistant to the development of destructive disease irrespective of the standard of oral hygiene. This leaves approximately 80% of the adult population to develop a slowly progressive form of disease that will lead to gradual tooth loss, particularly in the later decades of life but which importantly is amenable to a high degree of control by oral hygiene practices. The figures are similar from studies conducted in elderly populations. For example, in a survey of non-institutionalised elderly adults in the United States Midwest, only 7% of individuals showed signs of active periodontal destruction, as defined by gingival bleeding on probing and deep periodontal pocketing. Another approach to assessment of periodontal status is by means of alveolar bone support, which is viewed radiographically. In one study, 87% of subjects had over 60% of bone remaining. Although such results are encouraging, there are two important factors to be considered with respect to the elderly, both of which are relevant to health care planning. First, the proportion and therefore the absolute number of elderly individuals is currently increasing in many Western nations (see Chapter 1). Second, for a number of reasons, more people are keeping their teeth for longer. Taking a slightly negative view, the highly susceptible group

developing early onset periodontitis will lose their teeth by early adult life and therefore constitute a persistent edentulous population. Thus, the majority of the elderly will succumb, with time, to slowly progressive, unspectacular periodontitis but which will have particular and significant consequences for the provision of basic periodontal and restorative care. The current pattern of disease leads to the projection that the absolute quantity of periodontal disease requiring treatment in the elderly will continue to increase until around the year 2010. After this time there is uncertainty as to how matters will progress as other factors may come into play. The story of dental caries serves as a good example. Some encouragement for health-care planners should come from the observation that the younger age groups generally now have higher standards of oral hygiene with low plaque scores, so that in due course disease prevalence should start to fall.

As a generalisation, the highly susceptible patient is not likely to be seen in other than the complete or partial denture status. The young adult patient illustrated by the radiograph shown in **79** is clearly destined to lose her teeth in the near future. It is difficult to imagine this patient retaining these teeth into old age. The highly resistant patient is becoming more commonly seen although the patient shown in **80** may be an extreme example!

The more common situation is a middle group of patients, succumbing to slowly progressive disease but for whom much can be done by means of basic therapy and institution of good home care.

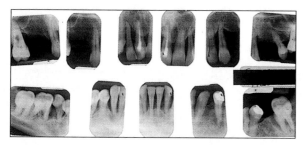

79 Periapical radiographs of a 34-year-old female patient, showing extensive bony destruction, despite 7 years non-surgical treatment.

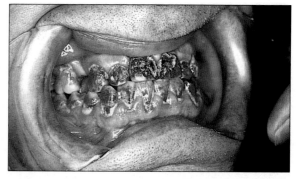

80 67-year-old man who admitted to never having owned a toothbrush. He presented to the clinic requesting a cosmetic cleaning prior to his wedding! Only one tooth was missing and there was no mobility of any teeth.

Figure **81** shows the upper anterior dentition of a 78-year-old female patient whose biological age appeared to be somewhat less than chronology indicated. She was a regular attender with a dental hygienist and her general dental practitioner and had only recently been provided with the fixed prosthetic bridgework seen in the photograph. Even when conditions favour the accumulation of plaque, disease progression is not inevitable **(82, 83)**.

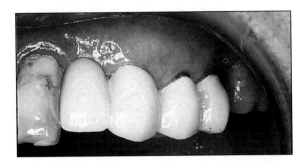

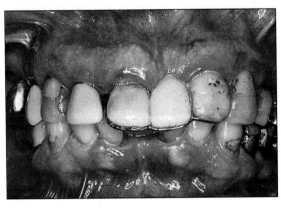

81 A 78-year-old lady who had recently been provided with fixed bridgework to replace the upper lateral incisor. Bone support and soft tissue status were excellent.

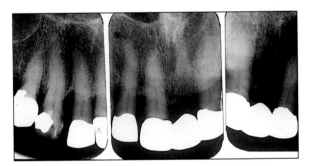

82 A 73-year-old lady with an upper anterior fixed bridge, fitted 26 years previously.

83 A radiograph of the patient illustrated in **82** showing that bone support has not been significantly compromised.

Periodontal problems in the older patient

It is important to emphasise that clinically significant problems that might be regarded as periodontal in nature are not the sole premise of the elderly patient, although some are more likely to be seen.

Periodontitis

As outlined previously, slowly progressive disease is generally related to the presence of dental plaque and a poor standard of oral hygiene. In the elderly this can be exacerbated by the progressive loss of manual dexterity, eyesight and more serious problems that may permit the expression of disease to come to the fore. Changes in salivary flow, for example, will also make plaque control more difficult (see Chapter 4). The destructive process is the same in all age groups, although ageing induces changes in defence systems so that generally there is a reduced number of circulating defence cells including neutrophil granulocytes and T-lymphocytes. The overall effect is to induce a mild level of immunodeficiency. Once again the process may not be significant but act slowly and in an unspectacular fashion. These changes in the immune system may be more relevant to immune surveillance with respect to the development of neoplasia.

Gingival recession

Becoming 'long in the tooth' has long been an aphorism for the ageing process and growing old. Gingival recession is widespread and, in addition to appearance, may concern patients by virtue of the ensuing root dentine sensitivity. However, once again, age brings its rewards and root exposure is more commonly painful in younger patients where there has been less time for the development of secondary and sclerotic forms of dentine (**84, 85**).

A more serious consequence of gingival recession is likely to be root caries and the dentist or hygienist must be vigilant in examining for such lesions during routine inspection.

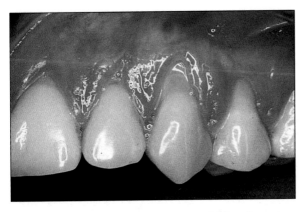

84 Upper anterior teeth of a 19-year-old female patient complaining of root sensitivity to cold.

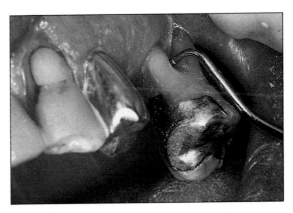

85 Extensive recession in relation to the roots of an upper molar tooth in a 67-year-old male patient. He had no complaints of sensitivity.

Tooth drifting and migration

With time and the progressive loss of bone support, teeth may drift and migrate under normal occlusal and muscular functional forces. This rarely creates difficulties with eating but may cause problems with access for plaque control. In the anterior part of the mouth such tooth movements may also cause concern about appearance (**86**).

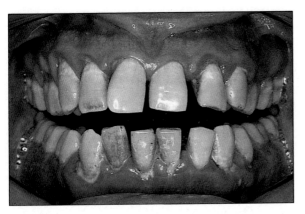

86 Drifting and spacing of anterior teeth in a 38-year-old patient with advanced periodontitis.

Traumatic root fracture

This condition, once unusual and rarely discussed in textbooks, is now seen more frequently. It is presumably related to the development of sclerotic dentine and thus a brittle root, favouring fracture by virtue of leverage at the bone crest. The problem is illustrated typically in **87**. The elderly male patient complained of sudden mobility of his lower right premolar tooth and the reason for this was clear on the radiograph shown in **88**. The fracture is clearly seen and there was little option but to extract both the mobile coronal portion and the remaining root.

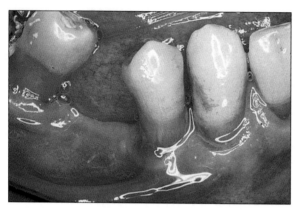

87 A 70-year-old male patient who complained of sudden mobility of the lower right first premolar tooth.

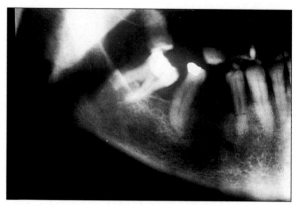

88 Radiograph of patient seen in **87**. The radiograph shows the horizontal fracture at the bone crest.

Periodontal manifestations of systemic disease

It is inevitable that the longer an organism is in existence, the more likely is the development of disease. This desease can be infectious, neoplastic, inflammatory, immunological or degenerative. However, to dispute the folklore and a common misconception, it has been shown that age in itself is not a determinant of periodontal disease (Abdellatif and Burt, 1987). Other medical factors may, of course, exacerbate the destructive process and a comprehensive account is provided elsewhere (Chapters 3 and 13). Some conditions deserve comment, for example progressive loss of neuro-muscular coordination will make oral hygiene practices more difficult, including the manipulation of tooth brushes and other oral hygiene aids. The problem may be particularly severe if there are additional specific disturbances of motor function such as Parkinson's disease and Alzheimer's disease (see Chapter 15).

The ultimate support tissue of the teeth is alveolar bone and this shows characteristic changes with age and sometimes dramatically so. The much publicised condition of type I (post-menopausal) osteoporosis may affect tooth support and this has been recognised in older women. It should not be forgotten, however, that elderly men are also prone to type II osteoporosis, which is less dependent on hormonal influences. Under these circumstances the loss of bone mass may be significantly influenced by deteriorating oral hygiene and thereby inflammatory activity.

Gingival hyperplasia related to the long-term use of phenytoin (Dilantin) for the treatment of epilepsy is well documented. A number of other drugs are now recognised as causing similar overproduction of collagen by fibroblasts within the gingival connective tissue. Of relevance to the older patient is the widespread use of nifedipine, a calcium channel blocker, which is effective in controlling simple forms of hypertension and is also used in the management of angina. In some patients, although not predictably, gingival hyperplasia will develop (**89**). This can be partly controlled by hygiene therapy but in some circumstances surgical

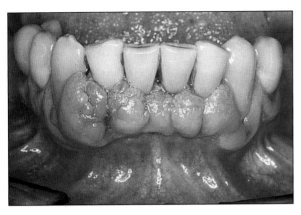

89 Gingival hyperplasia in a 57-year-old male patient taking long-term nifedipine for the treatment of hypertension.

reduction by gingivectomy will improve access for plaque control and also improve the patient's self esteem regarding appearance. There is no specific contraindication to surgical treatment, although the patient must obviously be warned of a possible and likely recurrence of the hyperplasia if the medication continues.

The prevention and management of periodontal problems

Oral hygiene

To reiterate the first and most fundamental point, it is the acceptance that whatever the role of the host response, plaque reduction is currently the main target for control of disease progression. The prevention of all gingival and periodontal diseases within populations, and especially in high risk groups, is no longer regarded as realistic or feasible but rather the aim should be to maintain functional health and, again, this is particularly relevant to the elderly population. It is therefore important to maintain a sensible perspective in determining prevention and treatment programmes for the elderly. Except in the case of sudden onset and severe debilitating medical illness, aggressive forms of periodontitis are unlikely to develop spontaneously after the age of 65 years. By definition, primary preventive programmes must commence in the younger age groups and then be maintained throughout life. In the elderly, realistic programmes must be planned. For example, in one study it was reported that 57% of the elderly patients screened had 3–6mm pocketing and therefore required root planing. A further 15% had pocket depths greater than 6 mm and thus required even more extensive treatment possibly including

surgery. Nevertheless, only 7% of the sample studied had bleeding from the base of deep pockets, a figure closely related to that for susceptibility in the population overall. Even in the light of the Random Burst Theory the question must be asked: how significant is 3–6mm or even 6 mm pocketing in an elderly patient and, therefore, what is the real treatment need?. Each patient should be individually assessed, but the approach should be conservative.

The maintenance of oral hygiene in an elderly patient is important and often crucial to the stability and functional health of the tissues (Abdellatif and Burt, 1987). Maintenance programmes can be highly successful and in the older patient will depend on manual and mechanical skills as well as continuing education and motivation from professional personnel, including dental hygienists (see Chapter 15).

Tooth brushes can be modified for easier manipulation, especially with respect to the design of handles (see Chapter 15). At routine appointments a simple plaque scoring system can be used to encourage patients by demonstrating areas that are being missed; these screening procedures do not require undue chair time. The simple scoring system shown in **90** is widely used. The presence of plaque at or above the gingival margin, after disclosure with a routine dye, is recorded for each tooth surface. The number of surfaces scoring positively divided by the total number of tooth surfaces available gives a percentage score. This can be used to assist patient motivation, although it has been argued that it would be more appropriate to encourage the patient by showing the percentage of clean surfaces rather than the percentage covered with plaque. Such an index has limitations, for example with regard to the quantity or specificity of plaque on a given tooth surface but can be easily combined with measurements of loss of attachment, pocket depth and bleeding scores.

In the United Kingdom, the 1988 Adult Dental Health Survey, although providing limited data on periodontal health and disease, demonstrated the importance of patients' self-care in the prevention and management of disease. This premise applies equally to older patients and especially where oral physiology is changing. There are also often local complicating factors such as the presence of complex restorations and fixed or removable prostheses. With the long-term maintenance of teeth in ageing dentitions, furcation lesions are presenting problems more frequently. These may 'smoulder' for a considerable time producing few clinical symptoms other than occasional bleeding but disguising the slowly progressive bone loss beneath. Often a simple surgical approach can be used to create better access for cleaning (**91–93**).

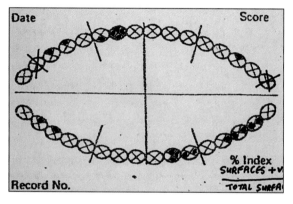

90 The simple plaque score record, to assist both patient and clinician in the maintenance of supragingival hygiene (after O'Leary *et al.* 1972).

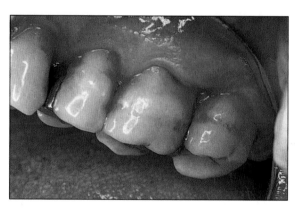

91 A buccal furcation defect on an upper molar. Marginal bleeding after probing is evident.

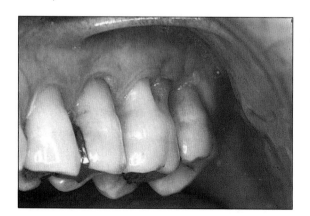

92 The molar shown in **91**, after tissue reduction and modification of the furcation (furcation plasty).

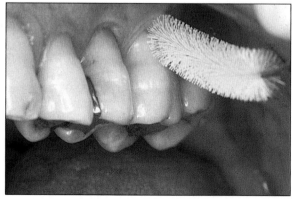

93 Compared with the initial state (**91**), the area is now more easily cleaned.

Dental hygienists have a particularly important role in this area of prevention and maintenance. In the United Kingdom they are now permitted to work with greater independence and, in particular, to undertake domiciliary visits in order to assist elderly or otherwise incapacitated patients. Responsible to the prescribing dental practitioner, they are capable of providing a major part of periodontal preventive care required by this patient group.

Antiseptic mouth rinses, particularly those containing chlorhexidine and fluoride, may assist in plaque control related to the prevention of gingival and periodontal inflammation and caries, especially root caries. Dentifrices containing antibacterial agents such as Triclosan and natural plant extracts are widely available although their efficacy beyond that of mechanical cleaning is generally disappointing according to the results of many clinical studies. Perhaps the exception is that of anticalculus preparations, where efficacy in controlling supragingival calculus is greater. Discomfort from root dentine sensitivity can be alleviated by the long-term use of proprietary dentifrices containing, for example, potassium citrate or strontium salts. More severe symptoms may require the application of sealant resins or bonding agents.

Periodontitis and the timing of tooth replacement

It is obvious that the need for plaque control is paramount, with a special emphasis in relation to restored teeth and fixed or removable prostheses. This is relevant in all age groups. However, one question often asked is 'when should periodontally involved teeth be extracted and then replaced?'. Clearly, one procedure does not necessarily logically follow the other, but the argument is often offered that the progression of bone loss, often supervised, will ultimately compromise the success of a partial or complete denture fitted later. It may be more appropriate to extract compromised teeth early and thereby, hopefully, preserve most of the remaining alveolar bone. Conversely, the presence of teeth helps to preserve alveolar bone and extraction leads to accelerated resorption, at least in the early phase. It is probably unwise to postpone the inevitable because adaptation to the wearing of prosthetic appliances is more difficult with time. Patients individually often have specific concerns about losing their natural teeth and equate this with the ultimate defeat and loss of self esteem. The clinician must therefore be sensitive to these various issues and adopt a flexible attitude. Figure **94** illustrates the case of a 64-year-old lady who positively refused to countenance loss of her last few remaining upper teeth. The radiograph clearly demonstrates an almost total lack of bone support although these teeth appeared to be functional,

The availability of osseointegrated dental implants now provides an additional option for the replacement of single or multiple teeth or to provide support for whole-arch prosthesis (see Chapter 12).

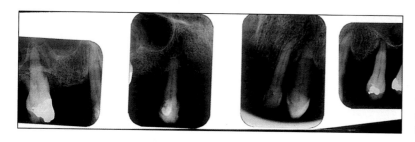

94 Radiograph showing extensive support loss around the upper teeth in this 64-year-old female patient.

Periodontal surgery

Until recently, conservatism and the lack of both knowledge and experience led to a guarded approach towards anything other than the most basic and simple treatment in older patients. An improved understanding of tissue biology has already shown that plaque control is more important to the maintenance of periodontal health than age *per se* (Abdellatif and Burt, 1987). It therefore seems logical to assume that tissue responses to surgical periodontics should also be predictably favourable, allowing perhaps for slightly slower wound healing in the older patient. Indeed this is borne out by clinical research in which tissue responses and healing after periodontal surgery have been compared in young and old patients. Healing proved to be satisfactory in both groups. This enlightenment should provide confidence in permitting the full range of treatment to be considered for all patients. Thus, treatment plans can be as realistic but also as ambitious as necessary. Some patients resist the extraction of teeth, particularly anteriorly, even when marked mobility is present. It may be possible to improve support through curettage and root planing and the placement of hydroxyapatite granules (**95–98**); after healing, the granules consolidated the base of the lesion and the tooth remaining vital.

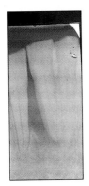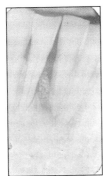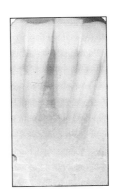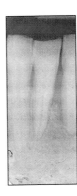

95–98 Four radiographs of bone loss in a 69-year-old female. From the left, the radiographs show the initial state (**95**), the appearance after flap surgery and placement of hydroxyapatite (**96**), and views taken after 6 (**97**) and 12 (**98**) months.

References

Abdellatif, H.M. & Burt, B.A. 1987. An epidemiological investigation into the relative importance of age and oral hygiene status as determinants of periodontitis. *Journal of Dental Research*, **66**, 13–18.

O'Leary, T.J., Drake, R.B. & Naylor, J.E. 1972. The plaque control record. *Journal of Periodontology*, **43**, 38.

Further reading

Douglass, C., Gillings, D., Sollecito, W. & Gammon, M. 1983. The potential for increase in the periodontal diseases of the aged population. *Journal of Periodontology*, **54**, 721–30.

Wennström, J.L., Papapanou, P.N. & Gröndahl, K. 1990. A model for decision-making regarding periodontal treatment needs. *Journal of Clinical Periodontology*, **17**, 217–22.

Genco, R.J. 1992. Host responses in periodontal diseases: current concepts. *Journal of Periodontology*, **63**, 338–55.

Levy, B.M. 1986. Is periodontitis a disease of the aged? *Gerodontology*, **5**, 101–7.

7. Restoration of Teeth

The decisions that are made as to what constitutes appropriate conservative dental care for the older patient must be tempered by medical, social, psychological and biological considerations that are related directly or indirectly to the age of the patient; these have been dealt with fully in preceding chapters.

Suitable treatment can only be planned when a diagnosis has been reached and a reliable medical and dental history, clinical examination, clinical tests and radiographs are essential requirements. However, it must be remembered that older patients are more prone to being medically compromised and have often undergone extensive dental treatment.

When a treatment plan is being formulated, it can be divided into four problem-solving levels, all of which are interrelated.

- Immediate stage. This level of planning takes into account emergency treatment for the relief of pain and the treatment of other acute conditions (see Chapter 3).
- Interim stage. The treatment considered at this stage is designed to interrupt the disease process and promote good oral hygiene. This includes the treatment of dental caries, periodontal disease and root canal therapy. It should also include a preliminary denture design so that restorations may be planned accordingly.
- Reconstructive phase. This stage is based upon the cooperation of the patient and ability of the dental surgeon and may involve the provision of crowns, bridgework and denture(s), partial or full (**99, 100**).
- Maintenance phase. This is essential for the elderly and must involve periodic review. It may include reorientation, remotivation and help with adaptation as well as further preventative measures.

Perhaps the most important consideration is that any treatment plan must be flexible and changes should be instituted as circumstances alter.

When considering routine conservative care for the older patient, treatment falls into four main categories.

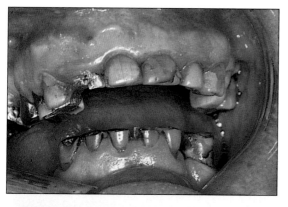

99 Example of a neglected dentition in an elderly patient.

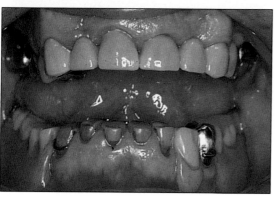

100 Extensive conservative and prosthodontic treatment restores aesthetics and function.

A. (1) Fractured teeth in the elderly

As more and more of the elderly retain their teeth into old age there is an increased risk of tooth fracture due, mainly, to the presence of large restorations which tend to weaken the remaining tooth structure. Loss of coronal tooth structure may be complete or partial. Cracks can develop which may or may not cause symptoms. Such symptoms may be bizarre and difficult to diagnose.

Masticatory accidents

These most commonly cause vertical fractures of the tooth and usually occur as a result of an unexpected encounter with an unyielding object during chewing, which is often very small. The small size of the object seems to be important as the normal proprioceptive reflex does not appear to trigger in time to avoid the object. These sort of accidents may occur in sound teeth but are more prevalent in teeth that have been weakened by caries or restorative procedures.

The effect of restorative procedures

The major cause of fractured cusps may be attributed to normal masticatory function applied to an already weakened tooth. The weakening results mainly from restorative procedures that have been undertaken in the past, such as radical tooth preparation during procedures for simple plastic restorations. Extensive cavity design for Class II amalgam restorations predisposes to weakness of cusps and this is especially true in maxillary premolars.

A major function of the cast gold restoration, as used today, is to protect and reinforce weakened tooth structure.

Overuse and improper use of pins

The injudicious use of intradentinal pins may weaken tooth structure sufficiently to cause tooth fracture. Pins placed too close to the amelo-dentinal junction may lead to subsequent fracture of tooth tissue in that area. If too many pins are used to restore the tooth this can result in weakening of both the tooth and the restorative material.

Previous root canal treatment

Non-vital teeth appear to be more brittle but the reason for this is uncertain. The moisture content of non-vital dentine is reduced compared with the vital tooth but this is probably not the full reason for increased brittleness. The preparation of a good access cavity for premolar and molar root canal treatment is, of necessity, a destructive operation and is usually carried out in a tooth that is already heavily restored. In addition, overzealous preparation in the coronal part of the root canal system may weaken tooth structure sufficiently to cause subsequent fracture. Over-enthusiastic lateral and vertical condensation may be the cause of vertical root fracture (**101**).

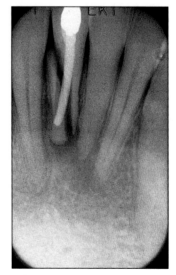

101 Periapical radiograph showing vertical fracture of lower incisor.

Excessive torque forces on abutment teeth

Inadequately braced abutment teeth of free-end saddle removable dentures may be subjected to torque during function, which may cause fracture of the crown of the tooth. Leverage can also be exerted on long-span bridges which may result in splitting of one of the abutment teeth.

The effect of intra-canal posts on root fracture

There is certainly an association between fractured teeth and intra-canal posts. Placement of posts may cause root failure. This is especially so with threaded tapered posts. If excessive force is applied during placement, the post acts as a wedge and vertical root fracture may occur. Posts that are too short relative to crown length allow enormous torque forces to be generated on the root during mastication (**102, 103**). This can result in vertical splitting of the root to the level at which the apex of the post was situated in the root canal, thereby necessitating extraction of the tooth.

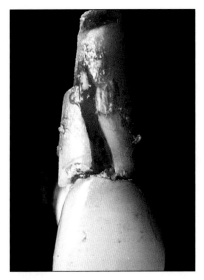 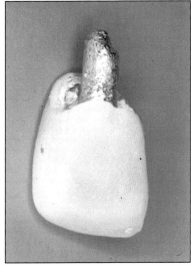

102 Vertical fracture of root as a result of torque forces.

103 Porcelain jacket crown with a short post can cause root fracture (c.f. **102**).

Trauma

Elderly patients may damage their teeth in any traumatic injury that involves the mouth. Trauma from the occlusion itself, however, may also cause cuspal fracture. Deflecting contacts between retruded contact and intercuspal positions on the inclines of vulnerable cusps, are particularly serious offenders.

Erosion and attrition may also contribute to the fracture of teeth in the elderly patient. The loss of tooth substance associated with these phenomena results in unsupported enamel which is weak and may easily fracture during normal function.

Dental caries

Dental caries is the most common reason for restoration of the tooth in the first place and it therefore plays an important role as a predisposing factor in the fracture of teeth. Caries that undermines cusps is especially notorious, as the weakened dentine does not provide sufficient support for the enamel. Secondary caries associated with existing large restorations in the older patient may contribute to horizontal tooth fracture with or without a vertical component.

Principles of management of the fractured cusp

Management of the tooth with a fractured or split cusp depends on direction of fracture be it vertical, horizontal or oblique, and the extent of the fracture.

Treatment of horizontal and oblique fractures of cusps depends, to a large extent, on whether the fractures extend subgingivally. It is possible to undertake periodontal surgery, with alveoplasty, to ensure that the margin of a restoration becomes supragingival. Elderly patients may not wish to undergo this type of advanced periodontal surgery and, if access to the fractured margin cannot be reasonably gained, then prognosis is poor. Other fractures can be restored using pin-retained amalgam, composite or cermet core restorations

and the tooth prepared subsequently for a cast restoration that will protect and support the remaining tissue. Where fracture involves exposure of the pulp, then root canal treatment is indicated. Non-vital teeth can also be restored with pinned cores or the root canal utilised for a post and core foundation.

Vertical fractures are difficult to treat (**104**). If a vertical fracture of a molar extends bucco-lingually into the furcation region then it may be possible to resect one of the roots and restore the crown. It could be argued that it may be less traumatic for the elderly patient to undertake this form of surgery than to have the tooth extracted.

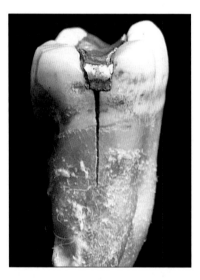

104 Vertical fracture of the distal root of a lower first molar caused by a masticatory accident.

Prevention of cuspal and tooth fracture

Large restorations should be checked to ensure that no excessive force is being applied during mastication and consideration should be given to protecting weakened cusps using cast onlay restorations. Forward planning in younger age-groups could avoid problems with tooth fracture in later years. Anterior teeth that need to be crowned should have a post of adequate length so that the torque forces arising during mastication are distributed through a greater length of root.

It is important that, during conservative treatment, consideration is given to the amount of tooth structure removed and efforts should be made to keep this to a minimum. The use of restorative materials that bond to tooth structure should also be considered.

A. (2) The cracked tooth syndrome

Enamel and dentine cracks are common in older patients and the classic symptom of cracked tooth syndrome is sharp pain, particularly on release from biting forces. This sharp pain probably arises from stretching and possibly rupturing odonto-blastic processes in the plane of fracture, and is often accompanied by extreme but fleeting sensitivity to cold or to sweet solutions.

The problem with cracked tooth syndrome is that it is sometimes very difficult to diagnose, especially if only a minor crack is present or intermittent sensitivity occurs, or if the patient has a high pain

threshold, and it may be confused with pulp pathology, temporomandibular joint dysfunction syndrome, and other facial pains. Later, the tooth may become tender to percussion but the patient may live with the discomfort for some time, learning to avoid eating on the painful side.

Finding the offending tooth is often a problem as the tooth may have been restored and the crack obscured. It is necessary, therefore, to use diagnostic procedures including tapping the cusps of the suspected tooth in different directions, wedging the margins of the restoration with a sharp instrument, such as a dental excavator, and getting the patient to bite on a rubber pad. Fibre-optic trans-illumination can be a useful diagnostic aid as light is not transmitted beyond the fracture line (**105**). If a crack is seen when trans-illumination is used, and is suspected of causing symptoms, a sharp explorer, which will often catch when run across the crack, can confirm its presence. Radiographic examination is useful to eliminate other possible causes of the pain.

Staining may be used to locate the crack if it cannot be seen. The restoration is removed, methylene blue sealed into the cavity with a zinc oxide and eugenol temporary dressing and, in 2 to 3 days, the crack usually becomes visible.

Many patients with cracked cusps also have moderately worn teeth and it is thought that patients who are clenchers or vigorous chewers are more likely to get cracked cusps, compared with patients who grind their teeth.

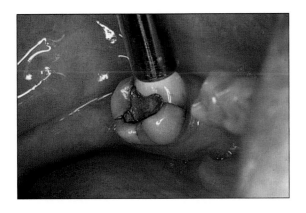

105 Trans-illumination showing presence of cracks in symptomatic molar.

Treatment of cracked teeth

When the offending tooth has been identified it may be possible to remove superficially cracked cusps and restore the crown. In some cases spontaneous fracture of the tooth occurs and the symptoms are relieved, except for sensitivity from the exposed dentine. Although 75% of cases of cracked tooth syndrome do not involve the pulp, in those that do, root canal treatment is necessary.

Cracked cusps have been splinted successfully with full-coverage gold castings and it also has been advocated that direct composite resin restorations can be placed in conjunction with a dentine-bonding agent.

Recently, a technique has been developed whereby amalgam restorations are bonded to the tooth structure using chemically active resins. Two such materials are Panavia EX, an autopolymerizing composite resin containing a halogenated phosphate ester of Bis-GMA and Amalgam Bond, a resin containing 4-META. The old restoration is removed (**106**) and the crown of the isolated and dried tooth carefully examined for cracks. A lining of glass ionomer is placed (**107**), but if the cavity is deep, then a sub-lining of a proprietary calcium hydroxide-containing material should be placed. The enamel walls of the cavity are etched in the normal way (**108**, **109**). Panavia Ex is then placed into the cavity as a thin wash, ensuring all enamel margins and the floor of the cavity are covered with resin (**110**), with amalgam being packed immediately into the cavity (**111**), and finished in the usual way (**112**). Long-term clinical follow-up of these restorations is required before they can be recommended universally, but in the short term symptoms have been alleviated and teeth have remained functional.

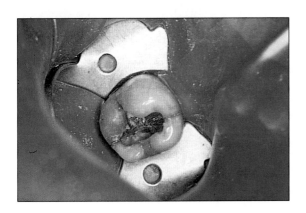

106 Mandibular molar with old restoration removed (c.f. **105**).

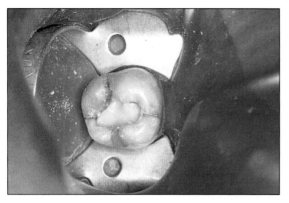

107 The base of the cavity lined with glass ionomer cement.

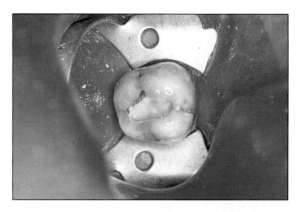

108 Enamel walls of cavity etched with phosphoric acid gel.

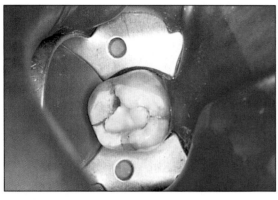

109 Typical frosted-glass appearance of etched enamel walls.

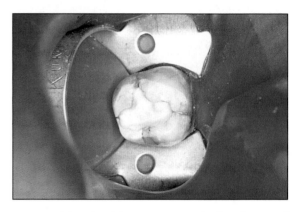

110 Freshly mixed Panavia EX applied to floor and walls of the cavity.

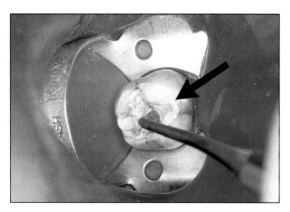

111 Amalgam packed into the cavity. Note extrusion of Panavia EX (arrowed).

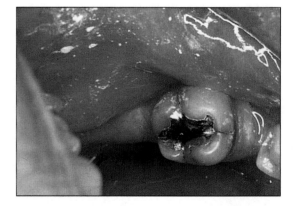

112 Completed amalgam restoration.

B. Dental caries in the elderly patient

As more patients retain their teeth into old age so dental caries is becoming an increasing problem. Many of these carious lesions are found on the roots of the teeth rather than the crowns, although recurrent caries around the margins of existing restorations is also a problem (**113**). The term root surface caries is applied to soft progressive lesions located on the root surface. Gingival recession, as a result of periodontal disease, is the chief predisposing local factor in the initiation and progression of the disease.

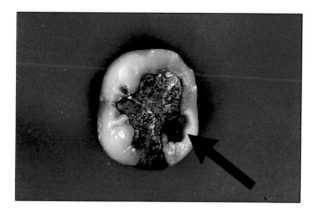

113 Recurrent caries at the margins of a large amalgam restoration in $\overline{6}$.

Root surface caries

The aetiology of root surface caries is poorly understood, but for root caries to occur there must be a susceptible root surface. It is generally agreed that the process is of microbiological origin, with elements of both demineralization and proteolysis. In addition, periodontally involved cementum has been shown to be softer than uninvolved cementum. The micro-organisms most often associated with root surface caries are *Streptococcus mutans*, *Lactobacilli*, *Enterococci*, and *Actinomyces*, including *A. viscosus*, *A. naeslundii*, and *A. odontolyticus*. Both *Streptococcus mutans* and *Lactobacilli* have been detected in higher proportions in the dental plaque of patients with root caries than in those with exposed root surfaces and no root caries. *A. viscosus* was implicated as the cause of root surface caries as, in early studies in animals, it was shown to produce root caries and periodontal disease. One group of researchers have suggested that *A. viscosus* may not have a role in the initiation of lesions but it may take over and dominate advanced lesions. The suggestion that a unique form of bacterial flora is present and initiates caries on different surfaces has not yet been proved.

Clinical appearance of root surface caries

Root caries is commonly seen as a soft, irregularly shaped, dark-coloured progressive lesion on the root surface or with undermining of the enamel at the amelo-cemental junction. It is seen more commonly in males than females. These lesions may be subdivided into active lesions, where the root surface area exhibits a darkened, discoloured appearance and has a sticky or leathery feel on probing with moderate pressure, with or without frank cavitation (**114**), and inactive or arrested lesion, where the root

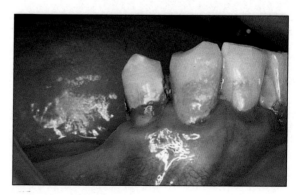

114 Active root surface caries involving the labial surfaces of $\overline{4321}$.

surface exhibits frank cavitation with a darkened discoloured appearance but is not sticky to probing with moderate pressure (**115**).

Active lesions may also appear yellowish or brownish in colour, while arrested lesions tend to be darker and often have a shiny appearance. Lesions may occur on all exposed root surfaces but are most commonly seen in the proximal and buccal aspect of the teeth, especially mandibular molars and premolars and maxillary canines. However, lingual surfaces of mandibular anterior teeth, in the presence of a removable partial denture and poor oral hygiene, are particularly susceptible in the elderly (**116**). Caries may extend to involve as much as one-half of the circumference of the tooth. Separate lesions tend to spread laterally and coalesce with one another (**117**). Patients do not usually complain that the lesions are painful.

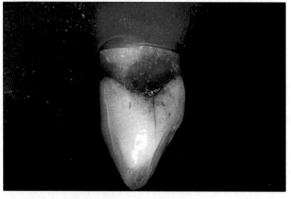

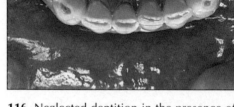

116 Neglected dentition in the presence of a partial lower denture.

115 Arrested root surface caries on ‿3⌋ .

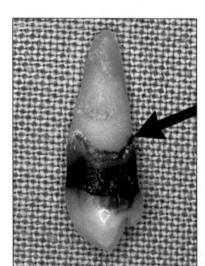

117 Extensive root surface caries in an extracted maxillary premolar. The level of periodontal destruction is arrowed.

Diagnosis of root surface caries

Diagnosis can be made from the clinical appearance of the lesion. In patients with poor oral hygiene the lesion may be covered with extensive deposits of plaque. The teeth should be examined when clean and dry and the use of sharp probes should be avoided. The presence of proximal lesions is more difficult to diagnose. Bite-wing radiographic examination should be used but care must be taken to avoid misdiagnosing the radiolucency created by the normal anatomic root cavity of the mesial and distal surfaces of the teeth.

Factors influencing the development and progression of root surface caries

Periodontal disease and oral hygiene

When the root surface is exposed to the oral environment, following periodontal disease, that surface is susceptible to dental decay. However, there does not appear to be a correlation between active periodontal disease and root caries. Older patients may lose some of their manual dexterity, making it difficult to keep their teeth clean, and are therefore more likely to develop root surface caries.

Altered salivary flow

Xerostomia or diseased salivary flow is a major factor in the development of root surface caries. Although various physical conditions reduce salivary flow, the most likely cause of dry mouth is the use of prescribed drugs (see Chapters 3 and 4). It is important that there should be dialogue between the dental surgeon and the medical adviser so that dental problems associated with the prescription of these drugs is fully understood.

Diet

A change in lifestyle in later years may affect the quality as well as the quantity of food intake. Retirement, bereavement or change of residence play a part in changing eating habits. There may be an increase in the consumption of refined carbohydrates, much of which is of a soft and sticky nature. There may also be a greater tendency to eating sugary snacks between meals.

Management of root surface caries

Treatment of root caries must be included in an overall comprehensive treatment plan for each patient. The principles of treatment lie in the management of active lesions by restorative means and prevention of progression of the disease process.

Active lesions

It has been suggested that shallow cavitated lesions may by recontoured. This is done using fine diamond burs, abrasive points, flexible polishing discs and prophylactic paste. The advantage of this technique is that it is minimally invasive but access can be difficult, especially interproximally. This procedure is accompanied by the application of topical fluoride. It is not necessary to remove all the stained dentine but merely to leave a smooth surface that is easily cleaned.

Gross lesions

These lesions with greater surface defects require restorative treatment and the material of choice is probably glass ionomer, although amalgam has been advocated where aesthetic considerations are not important. Composite resin, combined with a dentine-bonding agent, with or without a glass ionomer base can also be used.

Glass ionomer provides an aesthetic restoration that bonds chemically to tooth surface through carboxyl (-COO) groups. In addition, it releases fluoride which is taken up by the surrounding dentine and cementum. The material has a high degree of tissue tolerance and resistance to plaque formation. Although few adverse pulpal responses have been reported for these materials, deep cavities, especially those where there is freshly cut dentine, should be lined with a calcium hydroxide-containing cement.

Cavities that extend subgingivally are more difficult to restore. In these cases, a proprietary retraction cord (**118**) placed within the gingival sulcus may be sufficient to prevent contamination of the cavity and allow restoration. Electrocautery may also be used to achieve gingival recontouring (**119**). Restoration of a cavity using glass ionomer cement is described in Chapter 9 (**194, 198**).

Clinical handling methods and performance of glass ionomer cements continue to be improved and a wide range of shades, including darker ones appropriate for elderly patients, are now available. The introduction of encapsulated materials means that more consistent clinical results can be achieved.

Composite resin, used in conjunction with a dentine-bonding agent, has also been advocated for the restoration of carious lesions on the root surface. The coronal margin of the cavity, if in enamel, is etched, providing a microroughened surface into which the composite resin can flow and, following polymerization, provides a strong micromechanical bond.

Acid etching of dentine with orthophosphoric acid is controversial, however, and a dentine-bonding system is usually employed in an attempt to get chemical or micromechanical bonding to the dentine. The composite resin is applied to the cavity in increments to reduce the shrinkage that takes place during polymerization. A recent clinical study has suggested that composite used in the restoration of root surface caries performs as well as glass ionomer cement.

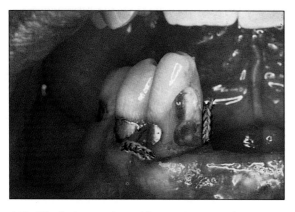

118 Gingival retraction with proprietary cord.

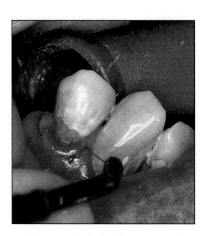

119 Electrocautery recontours the gingival tissues around ‾4⌉ to allow adequate access to margins of the cavity.

Prevention of root surface caries

It is important to protect susceptible root surfaces from decay. This can be achieved by instituting a preventive regime tailored for each patient (see Chapter 6). Restorative measures should be followed up with an intensive preventive programme to reduce the possibility of recurrence (**120, 121**).

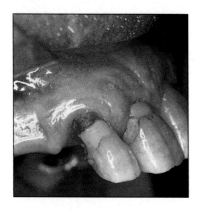 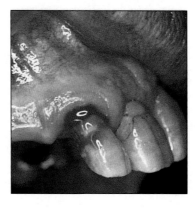

120 Arrested root surface caries on labial surface of 2⌋ .

121 Application of topical fluoride varnish to susceptible root surface.

C. Root canal therapy in the elderly

Acceptance of the social and psychological benefits of avoiding extractions has had the result that root canal therapy for the older patient is an increasingly important aspect of conservative dental care.

When considering root canal therapy for the elderly patient, problems can be encountered as a result of changes in the pulp chamber, or from the compromised health of the patient, or from both. In addition to the normal generalised ageing processes of the pulp (see Chapter 4), the tooth of an elderly person may have a history of caries, repeated dental procedures and restorations, periodontal disease and non-carious tooth surface loss. The longer a tooth remains functional, the greater will be the stress to which the pulp is subjected – the net effect of which tends to be cumulative and irreversible. As a result, root canal therapy on such patients tends to be more difficult than in younger age groups. However, complete obliteration of the canal space is rare (**122, 123**).

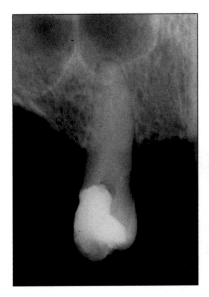 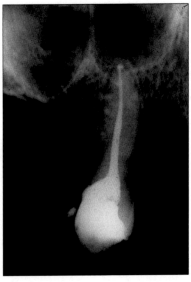

122 Periapical radiograph of 5⌋ showing apparent obliteration of the root canal.

123 Tooth successfully root treated (cf. **122**).

Diagnosis and treatment planning

The clinical examination must include appropriate radiographs. Mobility of the teeth and any sinus tracts must be noted. Bearing in mind the high incidence of periodontal disease in the elderly, the chances of a true combined periodontal/endodontic lesion is greater in old age. Such teeth have a poorer prognosis than those where the periodontal problem is superimposed on a primary endodontic lesion (**124**).

Most pulp disease is chronic rather than acute. Only when advanced pulpal pathosis affects the periradicular tissues can the painful tooth be readily identified by the patient. Until this happens, pain may radiate and be non-specific but, unfortunately, lack of pain does not mean lack of pathology. The management of and prognosis for root canal therapy may be altered significantly by the patient's medical

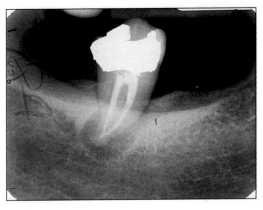

124 Periapical radiograph of a true combined endodontic–periodontal lesion of 7⌋.

history and concomitant drug therapy may have compromised the vascular integrity, neurological or inflammatory responses of the pulp.

Early detection of endodontic problems is difficult, relying as it does on an exact history of the pain being elicited from the elderly patient. The value of testing for pulp vitality with electrical or thermal stimuli is also reduced by extensive coronal restorations and reparative dentine deposition.

A change in tooth colour relative to adjacent teeth may indicate pulp necrosis, but a test cavity or specific local anaesthesia may be necessary to determine the need for root canal therapy in elderly teeth.

The full veneer gold crown or gold onlay may be appropriate restorations to protect cusps from fracture, thereby increasing longevity of elderly teeth, but the cumulative effect of previous insults to the pulp must be considered and over-preparation avoided. If a reasonable degree of doubt exists regarding the prognosis for such a compromised pulp, root canal therapy should be considered prior to any but the simplest of restorations.

Well-developed, undistorted radiographs are indispensable, to give an indication of possible problems which may be avoided or minimised, but these are not always easily achieved. A tendency for the apical section of a very fine root canal to be undetectable radiographically should not be confused with the not-dissimilar radiographic appearance of a branching canal. Magnification is extremely useful in studying radiographs of fine root canals (**125**).

Chronic pulpitis, often symptomless, may be associated with the increased apical radiopacity of condensing osteitis (**126**), or with apical radiolucency and loss of the lamina dura. Ideally, such conditions should be treated endodontically. A healthy elderly person is able to undergo such treatment but perhaps not if less fit, when a compromise may be preferable. Such a situation could occur in the debilitated elderly patient where the tooth is symptomless, useful and requiring only simple restoration. The decision to leave and review should be recorded and the tooth regularly monitored radiographically on the understanding that a worsening of the periapical pathology would necessitate extraction (**127**).

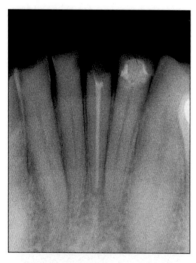

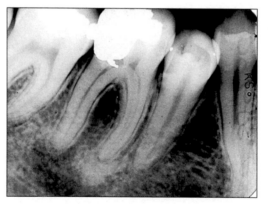

126 Periapical radiograph of 6͞| showing condensing osteitis associated with mesial root.

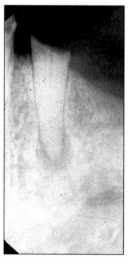

125 Periapical radiograph showing fine root canal anatomy apically from |2͞ .

127 Periapical radiograph shows |4͞ with an associated periapical radiolucency.

Pulp capping in the elderly

Pulp capping, or vital pulp therapy, is seldom justified in the elderly, as optimal conditions in the pulp conducive to its continued vitality and to the formation of a calcific barrier are not normally present. The success rate recorded for pulp capping in molars is extremely variable but is probably not sufficiently high to be justified as a satisfactory alternative to root canal therapy in a tooth selected for advanced restorative procedures. The exception may be a tooth pulp capped many years previously, with no radiographic or symptomatic reasons to arouse suspicion regarding the integrity of the pulp.

Reasons for considering endodontics as a means for retaining teeth in the elderly

Medical history

Endodontics avoids the need for tooth extraction and, purely on medical grounds, this may be important.

It has been shown that the risk of bacteraemia is greatly reduced. In cases where there is a history of rheumatic fever, congenital valvular disease or prosthetic heart valve replacement, endodontic therapy or restorative procedures involving possible gingival trauma should be carried out under an appropriate antibiotic cover.

For patients on anticoagulant or long-term steroid therapy, radiotherapy or with a history of high blood pressure or diabetes, root canal therapy may be the treatment of choice. For the terminally ill old patient in pain, this form of treatment may be less traumatic both physically and emotionally than tooth extraction.

Overdentures and partial dentures with free-end saddles

In come cases where considerable secondary dentine has been laid down in the pulp chamber, the decoronation of a tooth for an overdenture may not appear to necessitate root canal therapy. Such a procedure, however, may have produced an invisible micro-exposure that allows the ingress of organisms. Periapical lesions may take time to develop and routine radiographic monitoring is essential where overdenture abutments have not been root filled.

It has been found that the most common reason for loss of abutment teeth subsequent to the provision of overdentures was that of vital teeth developing periapical lesions.

There are important reasons for saving a mandibular molar whose pulp has become damaged irreversibly (p. 91,**124**) to avoid the need for a free-end saddle denture. The saddle of such a denture may be responsible for tissue damage and, in addition, adaptation to such a denture may prove difficult for the older patient. It is important that the long-term view rather than the short-term expedient should be considered and, in certain cases, root filling rather than extraction be carried out.

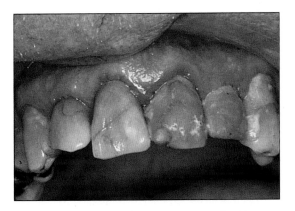

128 Extensive plaque deposits associated with composite resin restorations in |1 .

Psychological

The negative psychological aspect of tooth loss in the elderly or geriatric patient should not be underestimated. Such people should be treated sympathetically and, if practical and appropriate, teeth should be root treated rather than extracted.

Where it is considered that improved aesthetics would be achieved by crowning but insufficient coronal tooth tissue remains, elective root canal treatment may be necessary to allow placement of a post-retained crown. Teeth heavily restored with composite resin tend to retain plaque more readily than those restored with porcelain (**128**). Provided the enamel is of adequate quality a discoloured root-filled tooth may be restored with a porcelain laminate veneer (**129, 130**).

Root resection after root filling may also be considered where fracture or periodontal disease has compromised one root of an otherwise useful molar.

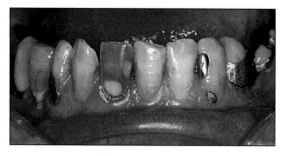

129 Root treated ⊤ in an elderly patient.

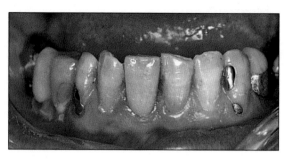

130 A porcelain laminate veneer was the treatment of choice.

Patient selection

The fundamental principles of sound endodontic therapy apply equally to all patients, irrespective of their age, local indications and contraindications being essentially no different. All caries must be removed from the tooth prior to root canal therapy and if it then becomes obvious that the remaining tooth structure cannot be adequately restored, such a tooth should be extracted. There are no statistically significant differences between success rates for endodontic treatment in different age groups, but the process of healing is slower in the elderly and large periapical radiolucencies may take some time to resolve. Where radiographic facilities are not readily available, root canal treatment may be inappropriate.

Properly managed, root canal therapy is usually well tolerated even by the rather frail elderly, but can be time-consuming. Many elderly, sometimes for medical reasons, find lying supine uncomfortable and, in some cases, distressing. This makes attempts at root canal therapy in most posterior teeth more difficult.

Root canal treatment

The reader is directed to specialist publications for general details of clinical procedures (see also Further Reading). The cases for radiographic assessment, the use of a rubber dam and an adequate access cavity are as strong for treatment of the older patient as for others.

Particular difficulties may be experienced with access (to a partially occluded pulp chamber) and with narrowed root canals. Both are more likely when treating worn or heavily restored teeth (**131**).

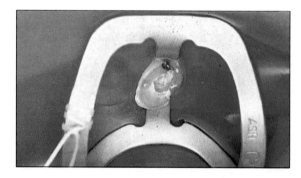

131 Worn anterior tooth showing straight-line access to the root canal.

Location and negotiation of fine root canals

Reparative dentine may completely or partially overlie the orifaces of the root canals. An endodontic explorer can feel for these tiny entrances and be used to pick away overlying spicules of dentine. A size 090 Gates Glidden bur may help to open up the canal entrances but on occasion a rosehead bur may be needed. In cases with complete obliteration of the pulp chamber, the operator must ensure that the correct path of entrance to the canal is being followed by taking several radiographs with the bur *in situ* and it is essential to look for extra root canals.

Single-visit root canal therapy

There are advantages to be gained from completion of root canal therapy in a single visit.

Although the single appointment may be longer, repeated attendance may be preferable for some old patients. In addition, there is a reduced risk of introduction of micro-organisms, which is especially relevant when vital teeth are being prepared for use as overdenture abutments (see Chapter 10).

Periradicular surgery

In the event of failure of orthograde root fillings, or inability to locate (or negotiate) a very fine root canal, consideration of apicectomy is not precluded. However, careful thought must be given to patient tolerance, and also the possibility that healing may be slower and complications accentuated. Additional care may be needed with pre- and postoperative oral hygiene.

D. Resin-retained bridgework in the elderly

Resin-retained bridgework has now become an important technique in the treatment of tooth loss. The use of bridgework retained by resin onto etched enamel was first suggested by Rochette in 1973. Since then a number of techniques, designs and materials have been developed and there are a number of long-term clinical studies that have demonstrated that this method of tooth replacement has a place in conservative dentistry.

The provision of this type of restoration should be considered as part of a complete restorative treatment plan. It is just one of several options, including full-preparation bridgework and removable partial dentures, that should be addressed in the reconstructive phase of treatment planning. Single tooth spaces are ideally restored with resin-retained bridgework, especially in the mandibular anterior region. It avoids the need to undertake extensive preparation of abutment teeth and thereby reduces both chairside time and cost to the patient.

Contraindications to resin-retained bridgework

There must be sufficient space to place the framework of the bridge without generating occlusal interferences and this can sometimes be difficult to achieve. Patients with a history of parafunctional oral habits should not be considered for resin-retained bridgework. The replacement of a number of teeth with a long span bridge should be approached with caution. A further problem with the elderly patient is the amount of suitable tooth structure on the proposed abutment teeth that is available for bonding, as many of these teeth will already be heavily restored.

Design considerations for resin-retained bridgework in the elderly

A direct pontic design using the patient's original tooth, or a pontic constructed from an acrylic resin denture tooth or composite resins, can often be used to good effect in the elderly as an interim restoration. They are easy to construct and provide a simple short-term alternative to the removable partial denture. The direct designs of resin-retained bridge have been largely superseded by the cast framework design.

A number of different designs have been described but a sandblasted fitting surface of the framework, combined with the use of a chemically active resin cement, provides a satisfactory restoration. Some tooth preparation should be carried out to the abutments to provide guiding planes and rest seats and hence resistance form. It is best to keep the number of abutment teeth to a minimum, as debonding of one of the retainers may not be noticed by the patient and leakage at the tooth–framework interface can predispose to the development of caries, which can be catastrophic if undetected. The use of a cantilever design is to be recommended wherever possible (**132, 133**). This design should be considered particularly in cases where the proposed abutment teeth have been affected by periodontal disease and are mobile. The fatiguing effect of torque forces acting on a fixed–fixed design of bridge in these cases leads inevitably to debonding of one of the retainers.

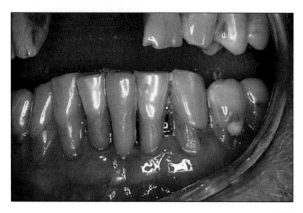

132 Labial view of resin-retained bridge replacing $\overline{1}$, which had been lost as a result of periodontal disease.

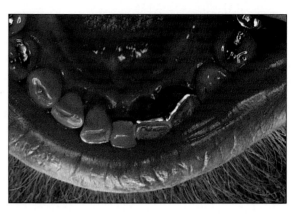

133 Lingual view showing good coverage of enamel by the metal framework.

Clinical procedures

Mounted study casts are necessary to help determine the proposed extent of the framework and the presence, or otherwise, of undercuts in the path of insertion. As much contact between the frame and the tooth should be sought (**134**) and, in the posterior region this can be enhanced by extending the 'wrap around' on the buccal surface. In the anterior region, the extent of the framework should be limited incisally to avoid the 'shine through' phenomenon which compromises aesthetics. Posteriorly placed rest seats are essential and should be spoon shaped.

Anteriorly, cingulum rest seats help give stability to the bridge as it is inserted. All margins should be left supragingivally but a compromise may be necessary in the elderly should an existing restoration already be present. In these cases, it is better to finish the margin of the bridge on sound tooth structure.

The presence of existing restorations in the abutment teeth may be problematic in that it has been shown, *in vitro*, that marginal leakage is reduced, if the bridge is cemented over an existing composite resin restoration compared with amalgam. It may be difficult, however, to justify the removal of otherwise satisfactory amalgam restorations.

Impressions should be taken in a rubber-based elastomer. The framework is usually constructed in a nickel–chromium alloy and the pontic in bonded porcelain. The fitting surface of the bridge is roughened by sandblasting with 150µm Al_2O_3. It is important that this surface should be protected from airborne contamination and so the bridge should be stored in water until ready for fitting.

The bridge is tried into the mouth with the fit and appearance being checked, as well as ensuring that there are no interferences in all jaw relationships. If the bridge is satisfactory in these respects it should be degreased by placing in alcohol, acetone or methyl methacrylate monomer for 10 mins. The abutment teeth should be isolated, if possible with rubber dam, cleaned with pumice and water and the enamel etched in the normal way.

The bridge is then washed and dried thoroughly. A resin cement is mixed. An example is Panavia Ex, which is an autopolymerising composite resin containing a halogenated phosphate group in its structure, which bonds chemically to tooth and metal and requires an anaerobic environment to polymerise. The resin should be placed on the fitting surface of the bridge and also on the etched tooth surface. The bridge is then seated onto the abutments aided by the presence of guiding planes and rest seats. Firm pressure should be applied to the bridge, on one side, and the abutment teeth, on the other, so that the film thickness of cement is kept as thin as possible. The margins are cleared of excess cement and these are then coated with a material to exclude oxygen (Oxyguard) to allow complete polymerisation of the cement. When the cement has set, the Oxyguard is washed off and any excess resin is removed from the surface of the bridge. Gross excess material is also removed from the margins of the bridge, but final trimming is delayed to a subsequent appointment a week later (**134–137**). It is important to check the occlusion to ensure that there are no interferences and it is essential that resin-retained bridgework is reviewed periodically, at least at 6-monthly intervals and probably more frequently in the first year. The elderly patient must also be given suitable oral hygiene instruction.

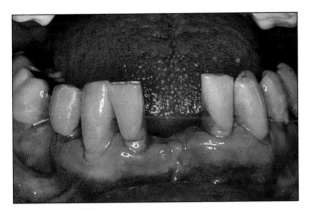

134 Missing 1|1 in a well-cared for mouth of an elderly patient with a healthy periodontium.

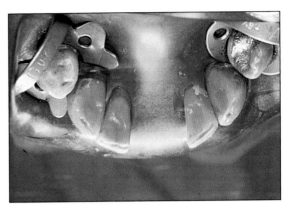

135 Rubber dam placed prior to etching lingual enamel surfaces of abutment teeth 32|23 .

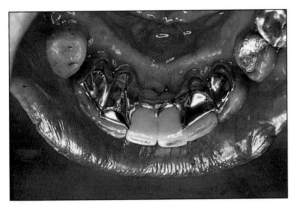

136 Lingual view of cemented resin retained bridge.

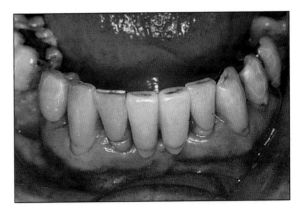

137 Labial view of bridge in **133**.

Summary

Patients are retaining more of their teeth into old age and it is important that these teeth are maintained in as healthy condition as possible. Good liaison between the dental surgeon, the patient, and patient's medical practitioner, friends and relatives will allow the most suitable conservative dental treatment to be undertaken for the patient. This will allow adequate function and aesthetics to be maintained to prevent difficulties in adaptation to dentures if teeth are lost in old age. Suitable preventive measures should be instituted early to avoid deterioration of the dentition as the patients get older and are less able to care for themselves.

Further reading

Banting, D.W. 1991. Management of dental caries in the older patient. In *Geriatric Dentistry, Aging and Oral Health*, pp. 163–4.

Crugers, N.H.J., Snoek, P.A., Van't Hof, M.A. & Kayser, A.F. 1990. Clinical performance of resin bonded bridges: A 5-year prospective study. Part III. Failure characteristics and survival after rebonding. *Journal of Oral Rehabilitation*, **17**, 179–86.

Ehrmann, E.H. & Tyas, M.J. 1990. Cracked tooth syndrome: Diagnosis, treatment and correlation between symptoms and post extraction findings. *Australian Dental Journal*, **35**, 105–12.

Kidd, E.A.M. 1989. Root Caries. *Dental Update*, 93–100.

Mount, G.J. 1988. Glass ionomer cements in gerodontics. A status report for the American Journal of Dentistry. *American Journal of Dentistry*, **1**, 123–8.

Mount, G.J. 1988. Clinical considerations in the prevention and restoration of root surface caries. *American Journal of Dentistry*, **1**, 163–8.

Newbrun, E. 1986. Prevention of root caries. *Gerondontology*, **5**, 33–41.

Saunders, W.P. 1989. Resin bonded bridgework: A review. *Journal of Dentistry*, **17**, 255–65.

Saunders, W.P. & Saunders, E.M. 1992. Effect of non-cutting tipped instruments on the quality of root canal preparation using a modified double flared technique. *Journal of Endodontics*, **18**, 32–6.

Thomson, W.M. 1990. Root surface caries – an overview of aetiology, prevalence, prevention and management. *New Zealand Dental Journal*, **86**, 4–9.

8. Conventional Bridgework

Tooth loss, for whatever reason, requires assessment of the advantages and disadvantages of replacement. Maintenance of appearance and function is an important consideration and frequently dictates treatment to provide a replacement. Although there are now several options including adhesive bridgework (Chapter 7), partial dentures (Chapter 10) and perhaps implants (Chapter 12), conventional bridgework is also a possibility (138). Surveys of fixed bridges provided by general practitioners in Sweden have indicated that, when well carried out, such treatment can be expected to last for some 10–20 years (139). Patient selection is, however, important. The question of cost and perceived priority for a retired person is obviously important. Perhaps more pertinent are matters of capacity for subsequent self-care and maintenance, and also the ability to tolerate the treatment process. It is also essential that there be consideration of the consequences of failure; even a temporary debilitating illness can destroy a previously stable restored state, as can an unforeseeable local failure (such as a root fracture).

This chapter does not, however, seek to give an account of the techniques employed in crown and bridge work but concentrates mainly on the common causes of failure of bridgework in the older patient, which should be considered when planning treatment for this group of patients.

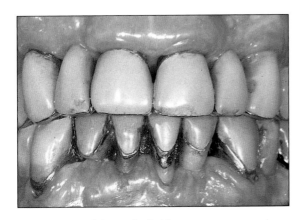

138 A successful anterior bridge.

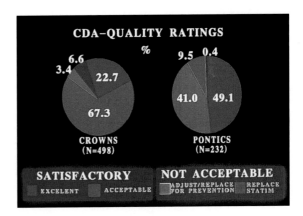

139 Quality of crown and bridge restorations.

An appropriate case for provision of bridgework

A typical case of an elderly patient is shown in 140 and 141. The patient possessed, for some years, single ceramo-metallic crowns restoring first and second premolars and first molar (140). Unfortunately, a root fracture of the second premolar occurred (141), requiring its extraction. 142 shows the situation after removal of the crown from the fractured tooth, and also illustrates a technique for removal of all-metal or ceramo-metallic crowns, using a slit cut into the crown from the buccal cervical

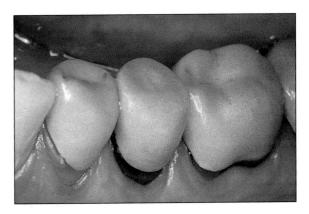

140 Single ceramo-metallic crowns. Root fracture diagnosed, second premolar.

margin. The cut is extended over the occlusal surface and then lingually. An instrument inserted into the slit enables the crown to be spread open with minimal risk of trauma to the preparation. After removal of all three crowns (**143**), the damaged premolar can be extracted, and the remaining teeth reprepared as abutments (**144**) for a three-unit bridge seen on completion in **145** (and radiographically in **146**).

In this type of structure, no significant additional distribution of sound tooth is needed (other than that dictated by the root fracture) and, indeed, the opportunity is taken to rectify deficiencies in the original crown preparations that had probably arisen as a consequence of gradual gingival recession (compare **140** and **145**), thus significantly reducing the risk of root caries.

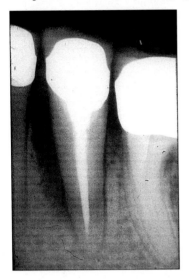

141 Radiograph of fractured tooth (see **140**).

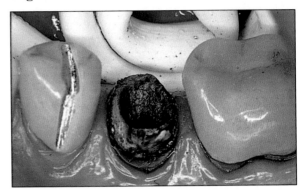

142 Same case as **140**. Crown removal in progress.

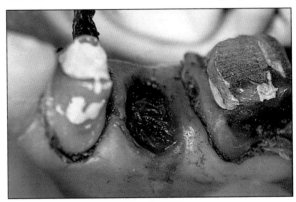

144 Fractured root extracted and abutments reprepared.

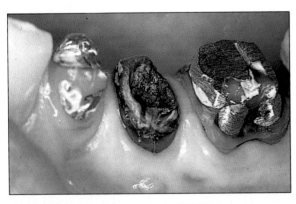

143 Completion of crown removal (**140**).

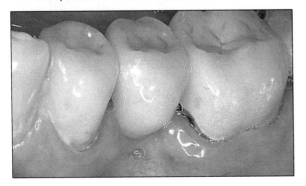

145 Completed bridgework (compare with **140**).

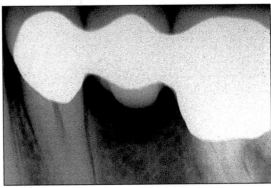

146 Radiograph of case illustrated in **140–145**.

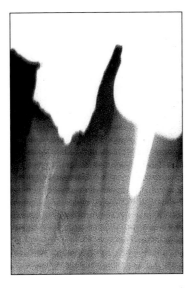

147 Radiographic evidence of secondary caries.

Causes of failure

Surveys of bridgework placed earlier have shown that secondary caries and technical breakdown are the most common causes of failure.

Of these, secondary caries (**147**) is the most common complication. Figures **148** and **149** show a case in which there was rapid breakdown of a premolar abutment tooth. The time difference between the views in **148** and **149** was approximately 2 years. Note that in this case the secondary caries is clearly visible. This is usually not the case; in other sites detection may be more difficult and therefore longer delayed.

Technical failure can take several forms. Early loss of molar teeth has encouraged the use of fixed restorations with cantilevered pontics to improve posterior occlusion. With this design, major stresses occur in the structure. It has been found that there is a linear relationship between the frequency of failure by fracture and the number of cantilevered pontics (**150**). Furthermore, the relatively frequent failure of such bridgework is time dependent – the

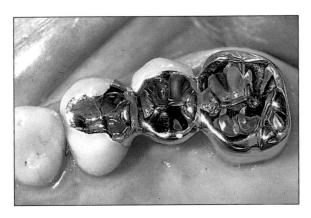

148 The original condition of a bridge.

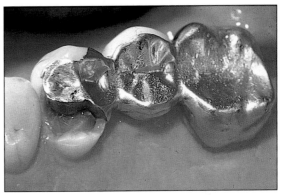

149 About 2 years elapsed between this illustration and that in **147**.

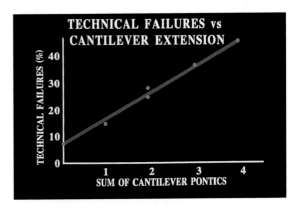

150 Failures of bridge structure dependent upon the number of cantilevered pontics.

101

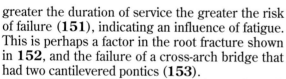

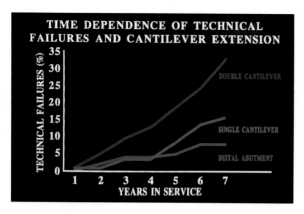

151 Bridge failures over time.

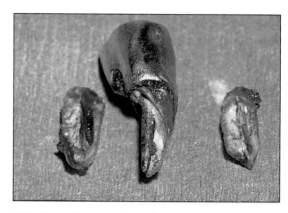

152 Root fracture in relation to post-retained restoration.

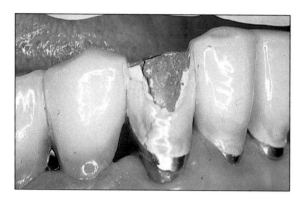

153 Fracture in a cross-arch bridge.

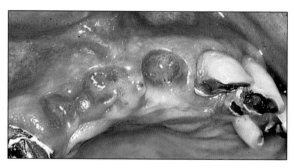

154 Secondary caries 2 months after detachment from the abutment preparation was noticed by the patient.

greater the duration of service the greater the risk of failure (**151**), indicating an influence of fatigue. This is perhaps a factor in the root fracture shown in **152**, and the failure of a cross-arch bridge that had two cantilevered pontics (**153**).

In addition to failure of the bridgework itself (**153**) there may also be breakdown of attachment to abutments. **154** shows the situation when about 2 months passed between the time that a patient noticed partial loss of retention, and the subsequent removal of the bridge. There had been rapid development of secondary caries on the abutment tooth.

In addition to mechanical failure of tooth structure, bridge structure and bond between tooth and bridge, there may be problems with tooth pulp and with periodontal tissues. Pulp death has been shown to occur in some 8–14% of all teeth subjected to conventional crown preparation, necessitating endodontic treatment (**155**), sometimes carried out through the occlusal surface of the crown (**156**) (see also Chapter 7). Periodontal complications are related to marginal adaptation and contour of crowns. Poor

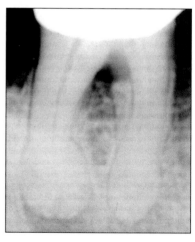

155 Apical evidence of pulpal pathology in an abutment tooth.

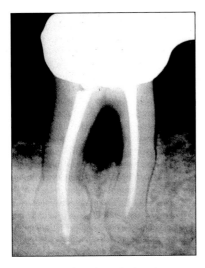

156 Completed endodontic treatment, using access through the crown (see **155**).

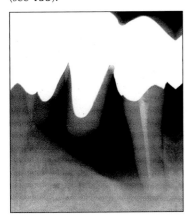

158 Advanced periodontal disease in an abutment tooth.

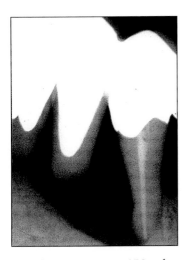

160 Same case as **158** after treatment and improvement in self-care.

contour and overhangs will almost always result in gingival inflammation (**157**). Well-executed restorations on abutment teeth, however, reduce the risk of periodontal problems to an acceptably low level (estimated at about 10%). In any event, such problems can be treated, and abutments retained. A case where even advanced periodontal disease was treated in association with improved self-care with respect to plaque control is illustrated in **158–161**.

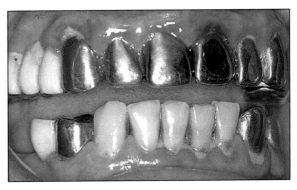

157 A localised gingival problem associated with an unsatisfactory restoration.

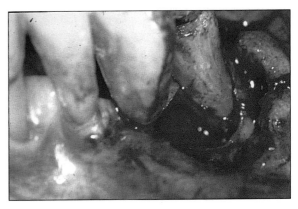

159 Removal of calculus (same case as in **158**) and curettage around ⌊4 .

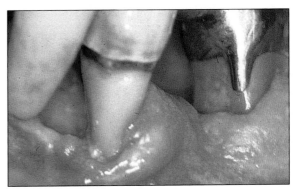

161 Clinical appearance after treatment (compare with **158–160**).

Selection of materials

The expected extended lifespan of fixed bridges requires careful selection of durable materials for their fabrication. Review of existing bridgework has demonstrated that acrylic facings are susceptible to rapid wear and discolouration. Figure **162** shows an extensive mandibular cross-arch bridge only 3 years after placement. A factor in this failure may be incorrect handling of the material. Another example is shown in **163** where there has been no obvious deterioration, in this case after 17 years service. In general, however, more predictable results can be expected with ceramo-metallic restorations (**164**).

Adverse mucosal reactions to bridge materials are comparatively rare, but there are an increasing number of such reports. Figure **165** illustrates a rapid mucosal reaction (possibly allergic in nature) to a polymeric material used to construct a temporary bridge contacting the lower lip, and **166** shows a delayed gingival and mucosal response to a dental gold alloy.

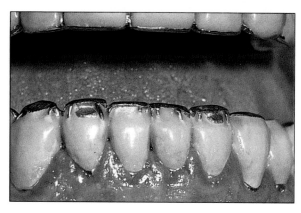

162 Deterioration of acrylic resin facings 3 years after insertion.

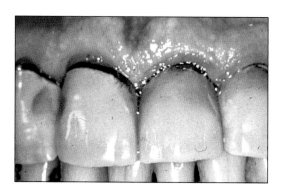

163 Survival of acrylic facings after long use.

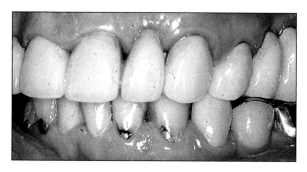

164 Bridgework of ceramo-metallic materials (compare with **162**).

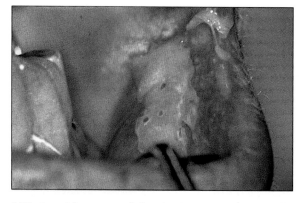

165 A rapid response following insertion of an acrylic temporary bridge.

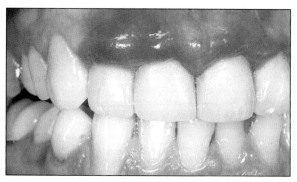

166 Tissue response believed to be to the dental gold alloy employed.

Further reading

Anusavice, K.J. 1989. *Quality evaluation of Dental Restorations. Criteria for Placement and Replacement.* Quintessence Publishing Co., Inc. Chicago.

Glantz, P.-O., Ryge, G., Jendresen, M.D. & Nilner, K. 1984. Quality of extensive fixed prosthodontics after five years. *Journal Prosthetic Dentistry,* **52**, 475–9.

Glantz, P.-O., Nilner, K., Jendresen, M.D. & Sundberg, H. In press. Quality of fixed prosthodontics after fifteen years.

Karlsson, S. 1986. A clinical evalution of fixed bridges, 10 years following insertion. *Journal of Oral Rehabilitation,* **13**, 423–32.

Randow, K., Glantz, P.-O. & Zöger, B. 1986. Technical failures and some related clinical complications in extensive fixed prosthodontics. An epidemiological study of long term clinical quality. *Acta Odontological Scandinavica* **44**, 241–55.

9. Restoring the Worn Dentition

Although by no means a condition unique in the elderly, tooth wear is undoubtedly becoming an increasingly common problem in the older dentate population. Several factors may contribute to this but probably the main one is simply that in these patients, the teeth have been exposed to the wear and tear of the oral environment for a relatively long period of time. Another important contributory factor is that many elderly patients are taking drugs for the treatment of a variety of conditions including ventricular arrhythmias, urinary frequency, hypertension and Parkinson's disease. Many such drugs cause dry mouth (xerostomia), which results in the loss of the buffering effect of saliva, making these patients more susceptible to acid erosion of the teeth.

Traditionally, tooth surface loss has three causes: attrition, abrasion and erosion. Attrition is defined as the gradual wear of tooth surfaces resulting from tooth to tooth contact. Abrasion is the mechanical wear of tooth surfaces resulting from an 'external' abrasive influence, while erosion is loss of tooth surface owing to the effects of acid unrelated to the carious process.

These three elements are rarely, if ever, seen in isolation and one of them will usually have the effects of one or both of the other two superimposed upon it. It is for this reason that the more general term 'tooth wear' was introduced by Smith and Knight (1984). The multifactorial nature of the condition is well illustrated in the case of a 67-year-old man shown in **167**. The shortened crowns and broad incisal edges suggest attrition; the loss of tooth substance cervically indicates abrasion related to tooth brushing, while the axial grooving seen mesially on both upper central incisors and the lower right central incisor is characteristic of acid erosion. The question that then arises is which, if any, is the primary cause of the tooth wear. While in many cases it may not be possible to determine what this is, there will usually be a single underlying cause and, if the most effective treatment is to be provided, it is important to find out, if at all possible, the nature of that underlying cause. The next series of photographs, therefore, will illustrate the clinical characteristics specific to attrition, abrasion and erosion.

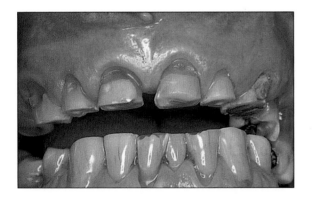

167 A 67-year-old patient illustrating the multifactorial nature of 'tooth wear'.

Attrition

The anterior teeth of the 60-year-old man in **168** have markedly shortened clinical crowns. The incisal edges **169** are broad and flat showing exposure of dentine and, in this case, secondary

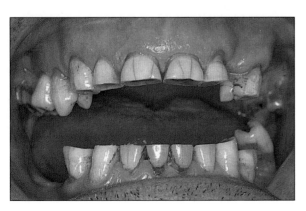

168 A 60-year-old patient with shortened crowns on upper and lower anterior teeth.

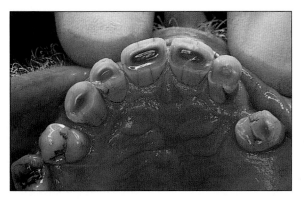

169 Incisal edges of upper anterior teeth (cf. **168**).

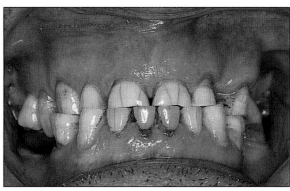

170 Anterior teeth 'in occlusion' (cf. **168**).

dentine. In contact (**170**), the incisal 'surfaces' fit well to those of the opposing teeth and, as exemplified here, the upper and lower teeth are usually worn to a more or less equal extent. Not uncommonly, as in this case, there are many missing posterior teeth. The fine microcracks in the enamel seen stained brown in these illustrations indicate heavy occlusal loading over a long period of time.

The very good gingival condition is another characteristic. This is often maintained, even with deterioration in plaque control as may occur in older patients and is illustrated in the 70-year-old shown in **171**. Exposure of incisal dentine is often followed by differential wear of the softer dentine compared with the hard enamel. This results in the cupping effect seen in **172** which, in turn, may lead to chipping of the incisal enamel shown here in the lower right canine and more extensively on the upper central incisors in **173**.

The aetiology of attrition is complex but is most likely due to a parafunctional grinding (bruxism) and/or clenching habit. This is often stress related but may also result from occlusal problems, including premature contacts and non-working side

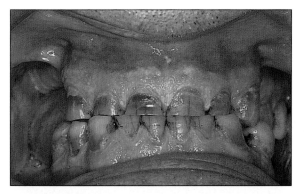

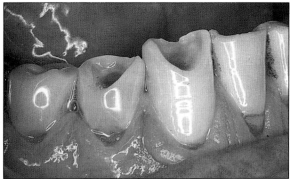

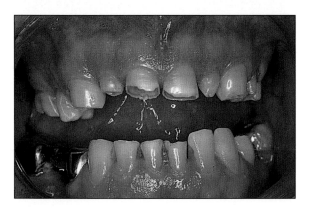

171 Ineffective plaque control with good gingival health (above left).

172 Differential wear of dentine compared with enamel resulting in 'cupping' effect on $\overline{43|}$ (above).

173 Differential wear leading to loss of unsupported enamel on $\underline{1|1}$ (right).

contacts in lateral excursion. Bruxism may sometimes be revealed by careful history taking. Traditionally, the loss of posterior occlusal support has been considered an important aetiological factor in attrition. While there is no evidence to support a direct causal link, loss of posterior teeth may be a contributory factor by inducing forward posturing of the mandible to give greater tooth contact.

Erosion

The clinical characteristics of acid erosion will depend, to some extent, on the cause. Thus, in general, if the source of the acid is dietary, the labial surfaces of the upper anterior teeth will be affected and, if it is gastric in origin, effects are seen usually on the palatal, lingual and occasionally the occlusal surfaces. There are, however, many exceptions to these broad generalisations.

The earliest sign of erosion, frequently seen first on the labial surfaces of the upper incisors, is a general smoothing of the enamel with loss of surface characteristics (**174**). This often progresses to produce the vertical grooving effect seen towards the incisal aspects of the upper central incisors in **175**. Early diagnosis is important because at these stages, steps can be taken in an attempt to prevent the problem by eliminating, or at least minimising, the causal factor. Any restorative treatment that may be required at this stage is quite simple. If allowed to progress, however, marked destruction not only of the labial surfaces but also of the incisal edges will occur (**176**). Note the increased grooving towards the mesial aspect, which also involves the incisal edges causing a notched appearance. This is characteristic of acid erosion.

Gastric acid tends to attack initially the palatal surfaces of the upper anterior teeth (**177**) causing

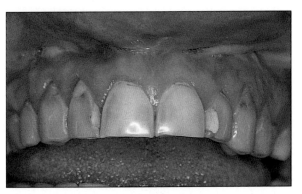

174 Loss of surface characteristics on 2|1 by erosion.

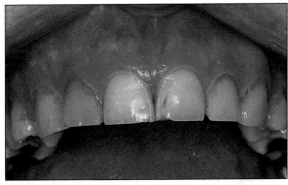

175 Vertical grooving of labial surface on 1|1 causd by erosion.

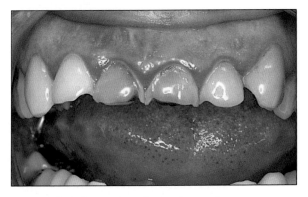

176 Marked destruction of 1|1 by erosion.

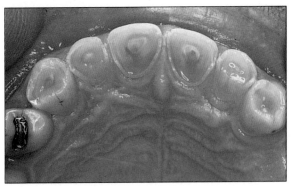

177 Hollowing of palatal surfaces on 321|123 from gastric acid attack.

109

hollowing out of the surfaces. It will also cause loss of tissue incisally resulting in shortening of the crowns, as seen in the labial view (**178**) of the patient shown in **177**. This can mimic attrition with which it is often confused diagnostically. The main distinguishing feature is that in centric relation, the lower incisors will not 'match' the palatal surfaces of the upper incisors. Indeed, they may not be in contact at all, although they often overerupt until they make contact. This has occurred in the patient illustrated in **179** who suffered from gastric ulceration over a considerable period of time. This shows the lack of 'fit' of the upper and lower teeth and, in addition, demonstrates that, ultimately, very severe destruction of the crowns of the teeth can result. Sometimes the palatal surfaces of the upper posterior teeth are affected, as shown in another patient with gastric ulceration (**180**). With teeth that have been restored with composite resin or amalgam, the tooth tissue will be dissolved preferentially, leaving the restoration proud of the surface (**181**) – another factor uniquely characteristic of acid erosion. Some patients indulge in deliberate gastric regurgitation from which they seem to derive some pleasure! This habit, sometimes described as chronic rumination, will tend to affect the occlusal surfaces of the posterior teeth as well as the palatal aspects of the anteriors (**182**).

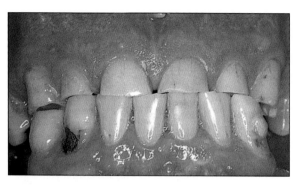

178 Shortening of clinical crowns in upper arch from gastric acid attack.

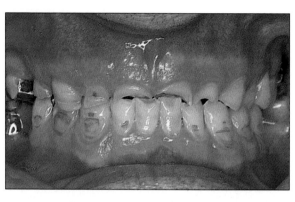

179 Severe destruction of anterior teeth with lack of 'fit'.

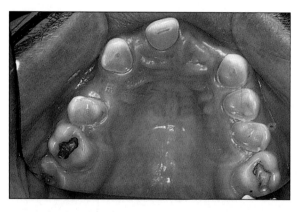

180 Palatal surfaces of posterior teeth eroded by gastric acid attack.

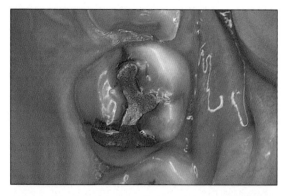

181 Amalgam restoration left proud of occlusal surface following erosion of surrounding tooth tissue.

182 Severe tooth destruction caused by deliberate gastric regurgitation.

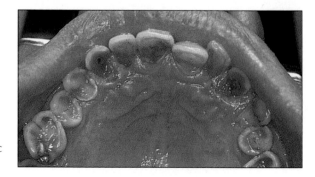

Clearly, in determining the cause of erosion, the patient's history is of fundamental importance. On occasion, however, it may be very difficult to obtain the relevant history. There are many reasons for this. It may, for example, be because the patient has difficulty in connecting a long-standing and perhaps enjoyable dietary habit with damage to the teeth, and therefore does not volunteer the information. Some patients are remarkably resistant to divulging information about unusual or excessive dietary habits. In the case of gastric problems, it should be appreciated that the episode that initiated the erosion may have been quite brief, not especially serious and may have occurred many years previously so that the elderly patient may simply not remember it. In all of these cases, careful sympathetic history taking, often with leading questions, will be required.

Abrasion

The characteristics of abrasion will depend upon the cause. Thus, **183** shows the abrasive effect of a pipe stem and is readily recognisable. The most commonly seen consequence of abrasion, however, is the so-called cervical abrasion cavity (**184**), generally considered to be related primarily to tooth brushing. While there is debate as to the true cause of this type of cavity, there seems little doubt that horizontal tooth brushing remains an important factor. Dental restorations, notably composite resin and poorly glazed porcelain, can cause abrasion to opposing teeth. This may be quite severe with ceramic crowns (**185**).

Abrasion is often secondary to acid erosion and may be the obvious manifestation of erosive damage. In **186**, the abrasion of the lower incisors

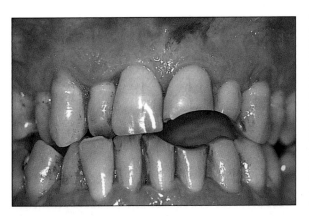

183 Abrasive effect of pipe stem.

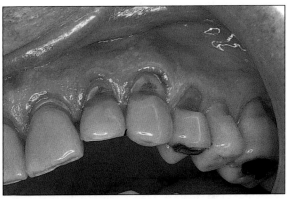

184 Cervical abrasion cavities on ⌊2345 .

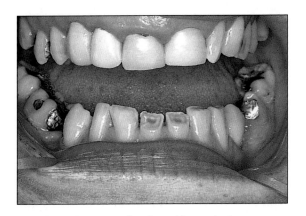

185 Ceramic crown abrasion of lower incisors.

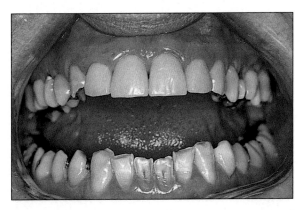

186 Suggestion of abrasion of lower incisors associated with porcelain crowns.

is apparently associated primarily with the porcelain crowns on the upper incisors. Closer examination, however (**187**), shows the vertical grooving especially evident towards the mesial aspects of the lower lateral incisors which is characteristic of erosion, suggesting this as an underlying cause. The effect of abrasion is the visible sign of tooth surface loss that can be seen in **188**. This degree of abrasion, however, could only occur if the enamel and the dentine have already been weakened by acid attack. This can usually be confirmed by history and the presence of other signs of erosion, such as proud restorations on posterior teeth. Progressive thinning of enamel caused by erosion results in yellowing of the teeth and may promote increasingly vigorous tooth brushing by the patient, often with particularly abrasive dentifrice, in an attempt to lighten them. This, of course, only serves to worsen the situation producing the severe effects seen here.

The cause of abrasion may often be clearly inferred from the clinical characteristics. If not, history taking will usually reveal this.

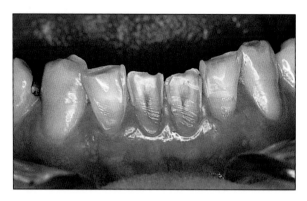

187 Vertical grooving present indicating underlying cause in erosion (cf. **186**).

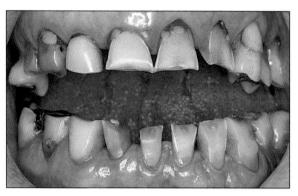

188 Visible tooth surface loss caused by abrasion.

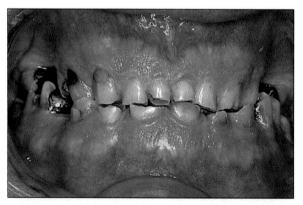

189 Long bulky alveolar process as a consequence of severe tooth wear.

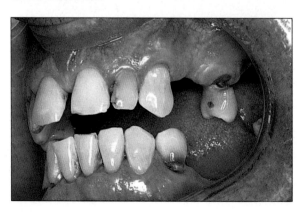

190 Dental caries in a cervical abrasion cavity of $\overline{4}$.

Other consequences of tooth wear

Tooth wear, from whatever cause, if it results in the slow reduction of height of the crowns of the teeth, is accompanied by progressive eruption so that the teeth continue to migrate incisally/occlusally together with the investing alveolar bone. This results in the long, bulky alveolar process seen in **189** and serves to maintain the occlusal vertical dimension. While the height of the clinical crowns of the teeth in these cases may therefore be greatly reduced, there will not necessarily be a concomitant reduction in occlusal vertical dimension. This may have implications for treatment.

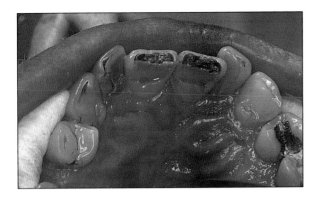

In the elderly, with diminution of oral hygiene, change in diet and/or drug induced xerostomia, plaque can accumulate in areas affected by wear, resulting in dental caries. This is shown with the cervical 'abrasion' cavity on the lower left first premolar in **190** and even in the cupped areas created by wear on the incisal edges shown in **191**.

191 Dental caries in cupped areas on incisal edges of 1|1 .

Management of tooth wear in the elderly

The first essential principle of management is, as far as possible, to remove the cause. Thus, if the cause is primarily gastric regurgitation owing, for example, to gastric ulceration or hiatus hernia, referral for medical advice is clearly required; from a dietary habit, an attempt must be made to change the habit while at the same time recognising that success with this approach with a very long-standing habit in an older patient may be limited. If so, advice that will minimise the effects should be given. A fluoride mouth rinse as described in Chapter 7, while helping to prevent caries, will also reduce the solubility of the tooth tissue to acid. Brushing the teeth before eating the breakfast grapefruit rather than afterwards, will help to minimise the damaging effects of the acid. This, together with the use of a soft toothbrush and avoidance of especially abrasive dentifrice is also essential if the severe damage seen in **188** is to be avoided.

Habits that result in abrasion such as the pipe stem abrasion seen in **183** may also be difficult to stop, particularly in an elderly person.

The cause of attrition is also difficult to eliminate because of the complex aetiology of this condition.

If there are occlusal interferences, however, these should be eliminated and defective posterior occlusion may be restored by the provision of removable or, occasionally fixed prostheses.

Having taken whatever preventive steps are possible and practicable and before going on to consider possible intervention, the question that must be asked is whether any active treatment is required. This will depend on many factors, including the presence or otherwise of symptoms, the patient's own concern about his or her perception of the progress of the condition, the appearance of the anterior teeth and the severity and rate of progress of the wear. In making a judgement on the need for treatment, the patient's age in relation to the extent of the tooth wear is clearly important. The patient illustrated in **192** is 72 years of age and, although showing significant tooth wear, the periodontal condition and the state of the dentition generally is remarkably good and clearly, apart from possible restoration of the cervical cavities in the first premolars, there is no reason to consider restorative treatment. In contrast, the patient shown in **193** is

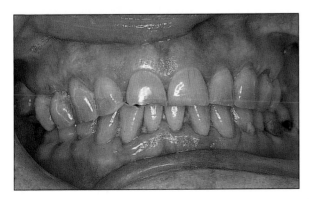

192 Healthy mouth in a 72-year-old patient requiring only minor restorative treatment.

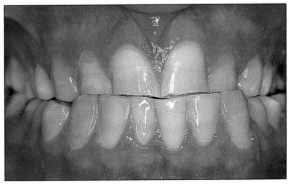

193 A 20-year-old patient requiring active restorative treatment (cf. **192**).

only 20 years old and a more positive approach is perhaps required in such a case.

Any restorative treatment of tooth wear should always be kept as simple as possible and the simplest type of wear to treat is undoubtedly the cervical abrasion cavity. This can be restored most readily with a glass polyalkenoate cement. These materials have the advantage in this situation of being truly adhesive to both enamel and dentine. They also leach fluoride which, particularly in the elderly patient, may be important in helping to prevent secondary cervical caries. Although glass polyalkenoate cements are relatively non-irritant to the pulp, it is prudent to line deeper cavities with a calcium-hydroxide containing cement (**194**). After insertion of the glass polyalkenoate cement (**195**), a matrix is essential (**196**) to ensure a satisfactory surface on the resultant restoration. After removal of the matrix, any minor finishing to the margins of the restoration may be carried out using flexible discs lubricated with petroleum jelly (**197**). The com-

pleted restoration, protected with a waterproof varnish, is shown in **198**. The relative lack of translucency of glass polyalkenoate cement may limit its use where appearance is of importance, as with large defects in the upper central incisors shown in **199**. Here, the laminate technique which combines the dentine-bonding properties of glass polyalkenoate with the enamel-bonding properties and superior aesthetics of composite resin may be used. The long-term effectiveness of these restorations is the subject of some controversy at present, but there are still clinical indications for their use. The basic construction of such a restoration is shown in **200**. The teeth are isolated with a rubber dam, where possible (**201**), and the glass polyalkenoate applied (**202**). There is debate whether the glass polyalkenoate should then be etched to provide improved micromechanical bonding with the composite resin but the balance of opinion seems to be against doing so. The enamel incisal margin of the cavity only, therefore, is etched (**203**), unfilled resin applied

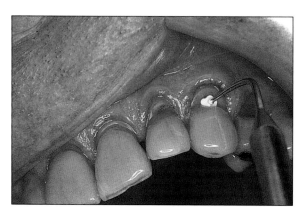

194 Placement of calcium hydroxide-containing cement in |3 .

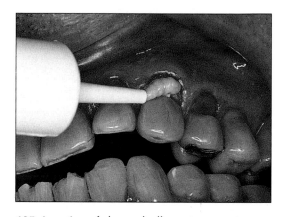

195 Insertion of glass polyalkenoate cement.

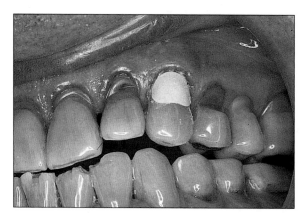

196 Placement of matrix over restoration in |3 .

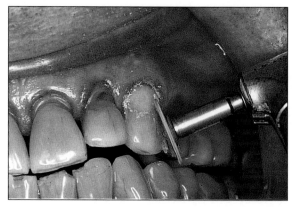

197 Minor finishing using flexible discs lubricated with petroleum jelly.

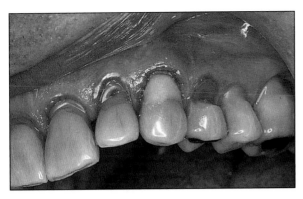

198 Completed restoration in ⌊3 .

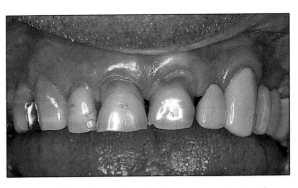

199 Consideration of aesthetics when restoring large defects on 1⌋1 .

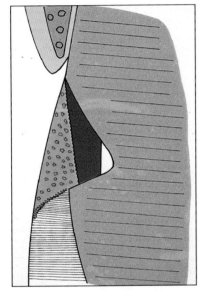

200 Diagrammatic representation showing restoration of a cervical cavity using a laminate technique.

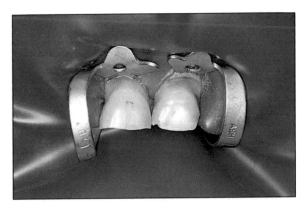

201 1⌋1 requiring restoration isolated with rubber dam.

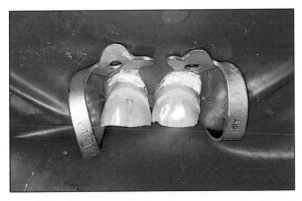

202 Glass polyalkenoate cement applied to cervical cavities in 1⌋1 .

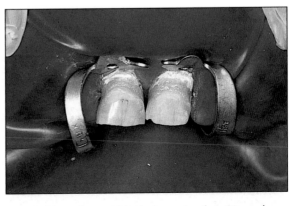

203 Etching of enamel incisal margin of cavities only.

(204) and the composite inserted with a suitable matrix (205). The final result is shown in 206.

In many cases, simple treatment may not be possible, as with the pipe stem abrasion shown in 183. Here composite restorations would quickly succumb so that traditional porcelain jacket crowns (207) have been used. Conventional crowning techniques may also be used where severe tooth destruction has occurred, as in the case in 177 and 178 and where the patient is both willing and able to undergo the lengthy clinical procedure required. Here an increase in vertical dimension was required and the patient's ability to tolerate this was assessed initially by wearing a temporary partial lower denture (208). Endodontics was necessary to allow crowns to be retained on the upper anterior teeth (209). In such cases when increasing the occlusal vertical dimension primarily by means of a partial

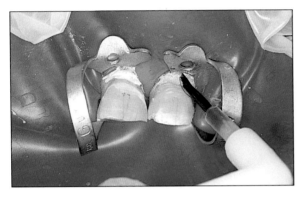

204 Application of unfilled composite resin.

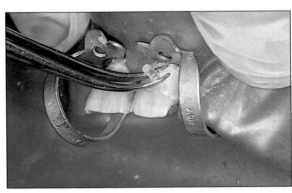

205 Insertion of composite with suitable matrix in place.

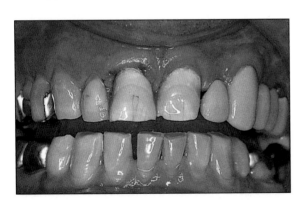

206 Completed cervical restorations in 1|1 .

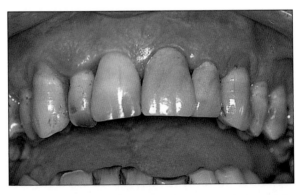

207 Restoration of pipe stem abrasion with porcelain jacket crown on |12 (cf. 183).

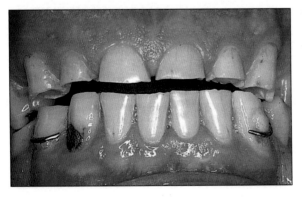

208 Provision of partial lower denture to assess patients ability to tolerate an increase in occlusal vertical dimension.

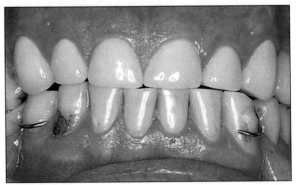

209 Provision of porcelain crowns on anterior teeth to new occlusal vertical dimension (cf. 208).

denture, it is important to provide a permanent occlusal 'stop' at the increased vertical height so that the anterior crowns will be protected when the denture is removed. The principle of the posterior occlusal stop is well illustrated in **210** and **211**, where initial assessment of the altered occlusal vertical dimension has been by a temporary clear acrylic appliance. The lower left first premolar has

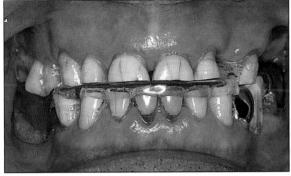

210 Provision of temporary clear acrylic appliance to assess toleration of an increase in occlusal vertical dimension.

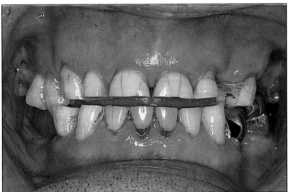

211 Provision of gold shell crown on $\underline{4}$ to provide posterior occlusal stop.

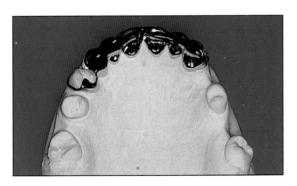

213 Provision of Dahl appliance to provide inter-incisal space.

then been crowned to provide contact with the opposing premolar at the increased height prior to crowning the upper anterior teeth and provision of permanent partial lower dentures (**212**).

In many older patients with tooth wear, there is loss of posterior teeth, frequently associated with loss of occlusal vertical dimension so that space for the restoration of anterior teeth can readily be achieved by the provision of partial dentures as described above. Where most of the posterior teeth are present, however, and therefore a partial denture is not required, the necessary inter-incisal space to allow restoration of the teeth can be achieved by having the patient wear, for several weeks, an appliance of the sort shown in **213**. This approach was first described by Dahl *et al.* in 1975 and the appliance is often described as a Dahl appliance. Only minimal palatal space will be needed if metallo-ceramic crowns in which the palatal surface is constructed only in metal, are used. Where there is an edge-to-edge incisor relationship, the metal can be brought over the incisal edges, thus minimising the amount of incisal reduction required (**214**). This has the added advantage that it will help to prevent ongoing wear of the opposing teeth.

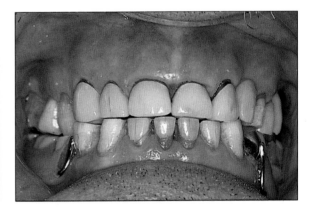

212 Completed restorative treatment (cf. **210**).

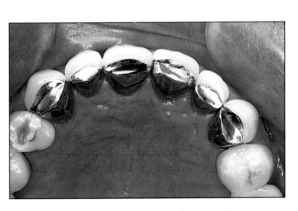

214 Coverage of incisal region by metallo-ceramic crowns in edge-to-edge incisor relationship.

One of the problems encountered in crowning severely worn anterior teeth is the lack of height of clinical crown available for retention of the restoration. While surgical crown lengthening procedures can be carried out, this is rarely indicated in an elderly patient. If the preparation for a metallo-ceramic crown incorporates a cervical chamfer, however (**215**), retention will be greatly increased. The crown is constructed with a narrow metal cervical collar, as illustrated in the constructional diagram in **216**. The tooth preparation itself is shown in **217** and the crown in **218**. This is the technique that was used in the case illustrated in **210–212**.

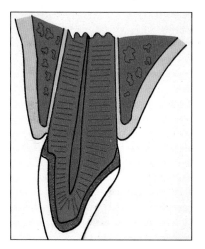

215 Incorporation of cervical chamfer in preparation for metallo-ceramic crown.

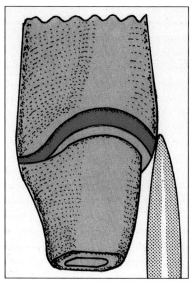

216 Construction of metallo-ceramic crown with narrow metal cervical collar.

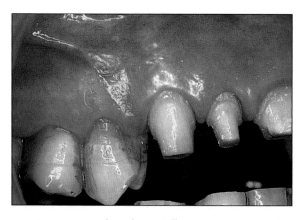

217 Preparation of 3⌋ for metallo-ceramic crown using cervical chamfer.

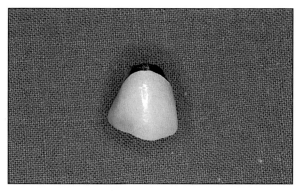

218 Metallo-ceramic crown with cervical collar for 3⌋.

Where teeth have been severely damaged in a mouth where a partial denture is either already worn, or is required to restore posterior occlusion, an overdenture technique may provide a much simpler but very effective means of restorative management (see Chapter 10).

Many patients, however, especially those in an older age group, are neither willing nor able to undergo the time-consuming treatments necessary for crown work or the multiple endodontics that are often necessary prerequisites to the provision of an overdenture. It is essential, therefore, for the treatment of the steadily increasing numbers of older patients suffering from tooth wear that restorative techniques are developed that are less complex, more conservative and less expensive than some of those shown and described above. In the case shown in **219**, crowns were contraindicated both by the extent of the tooth destruction and the age of the patient. Because of the palatal wear and consequent staining of the dentine, the labial appearance of the upper anterior teeth was poor (**220**). After provision of a partial denture, nickel–chrome palatal veneers (**221**), together with ceramic labial veneers (**222**) were used to restore the four upper incisors. The metal palatal veneers can be effectively bonded using a chemically active resin such as Panavia. An even more conservative approach was taken with a 75-year-old lady in **223** who was suffering from continuing sensitivity of the upper central incisors as a result of severe tooth wear related to gastric regurgitation many years previously. After provision of a partial upper denture (not shown) to give a slight increase in occlusal dimension, the upper central incisors were restored with laboratory-cured resin palatal veneers (**224**). These were continued over the

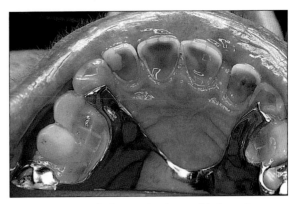

219 Anterior tooth destruction in an elderly patient.

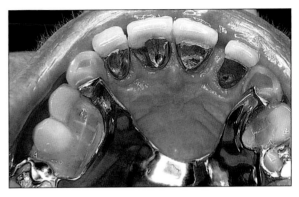

221 Provision of nickel–chrome veneers to palatal surfaces of anterior teeth (cf. **219**).

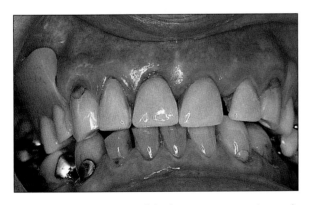

220 Labial appearance of anterior teeth (cf. **219**).

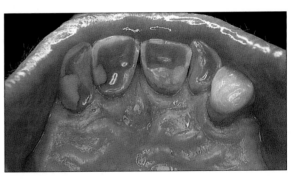

223 Loss of tooth substance as a result of severe tooth wear.

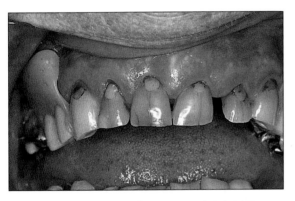

222 Provision of ceramic labial veneers to anterior teeth (cf. **220**).

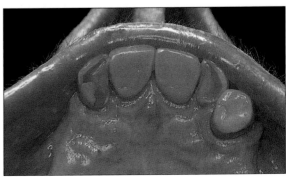

224 Provision of laboratory-cured resin palatal veneers on 1|1 .

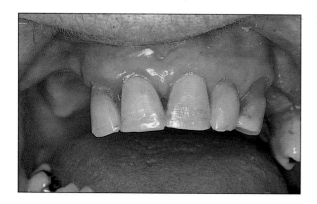

225 Palatal veneers continued over incisal edge to give improvement in labial appearance of 1|1 (cf. 223).

incisal edge to give a marked improvement in labial appearance (225). Note that in this case, the permanent stop has been provided by a similar resin onlay restoration on the upper left canine, constructed to give broad contact with the opposing tooth. While possibly less permanent than the metal/ceramic veneer combination, this approach has the merits of conservation and simplicity – principles that must be applied wherever possible in planning of restorative dental treatment for our elderly patients.

References

Dahl, B.L., Krogstad, O. & Karlsen, K. 1975. An alternative treatment in cases with advanced localized attrition. *Journal of Oral Rehabilitation* 2, 209–14.

Smith, B.G.N. & Knight J.K. 1984a. An index for measuring the wear of teeth. *British Dental Journal*, 156, 435–8.

Smith, B.G.N. & Knight J.K. 1984b. A comparison of tooth wear with aetiological factors. *British Dental Journal*, 157, 16.

Further reading

Eccles, J.D. 1982. Tooth surface loss from abrasion, attrition and erosion. *Dental Update,* 9, 363–74; 376–8; 380–1.

10. The Partially Dentate Patient: Removable Prosthodontics

Suitable partial dentures can be defined as dentures that are acceptable to the patient, that fulfil the functions they are designed for, such as improving appearance or masticatory function, and minimise damage to the remaining teeth and the associated soft tissue.

These requirements can only be met by adopting a logical sequence of patient assessment, the use of study casts for design and, perhaps most important, discussion with the patient before carrying out the treatment.

The initial consideration is the patient's attitude to being provided with partial dentures. In the elderly patient, there may be a desire for dentures to improve appearance, help with eating and reduce the wear on natural teeth. Conversely, partial dentures may be considered a waste of time, and the patient may request extractions of all the remaining teeth.

The next consideration is the patient's dentition. It is the biological age of the dentition that is most important rather than the biological age of the patient (**226, 227**).

Oversimplification in assessing the patient's needs is to be avoided but classifying the dentitions of these patients into broad categories is helpful for discussion and treatment planning.

The first category of dentition is a reasonable number of sound teeth with healthy supporting tissue where the prospect of further tooth loss within a 5-year period is slight.

A second category of dentition is where the teeth are either fewer in number or less sound, especially from the point of view of their periodontal support, and where the prospect of further tooth loss within 5 years is considerable.

A third category of dentition is where some of the teeth are so diseased either from caries or periodontal disease that the initial treatment plan will include an immediate partial denture or extraction of some teeth and the provision of partial dentures after healing.

A fourth category of dentition is where there are problems caused by loss of tooth tissue, drifting and tilting of teeth, an uneven distribution of teeth between the upper and lower jaw, especially if more teeth are present in the upper jaw, and perhaps a history of difficulties with previous conventional partial dentures.

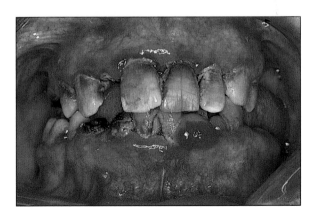

226 Poor dentition. Female aged 61 years.

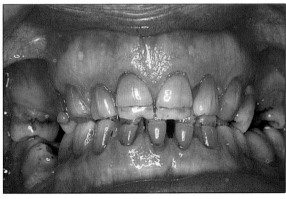

227 Good dentition despite mottling. Female aged 74 years.

Clinical examination

The clinical examination (**228**) must be supported by obtaining study casts (**229**), any necessary radiographs and other diagnostic measures. The importance of surveyed study casts is to allow the practitioner to examine occlusal relationships, undercuts suitable for retention by clasps, tissue undercuts, and the distance from gingival crevice. In fact, all the information that is required for sensible prescription for partial dentures.

The clinical examination and all the information from the study casts allow a treatment plan, including the prescription for partial dentures, to be developed.

The next stage is to discuss this plan with the patient. It may be found that the patient wishes only one denture, does not like the idea of clasps, prefers acrylic plates to metal bars, or finds the cost prohibitive. However, in most cases, a well-prepared treatment plan will be accepted by the patient. The author's view is that if a sensible compromise between practitioner and patient cannot be reached, then the patient should be advised to seek treatment elsewhere.

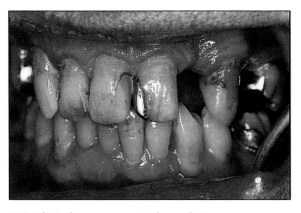

228 Clinical appearance. Male aged 66 years.

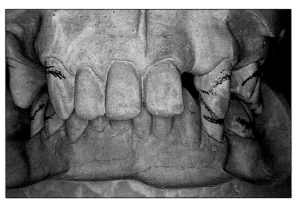

229 Study casts surveyed. Case shown in **228**.

Design considerations

At the beginning of this chapter the importance of the biological age of the dentition was stressed and a simple classification of the elderly dentition was described. The relationship between the clinical pictures defined by the classification and sensible partial denture designs will now be discussed.

In the first category (**230**) the dentition consists of a reasonable number of healthy teeth and good prospects for the long-term retention of these teeth. In these circumstances, the indications are for the provision of a metal bar as the connector. The standing teeth are used to support the denture by the use of occlusal and cingulum coverage and to provide retention by using suitable clasps.

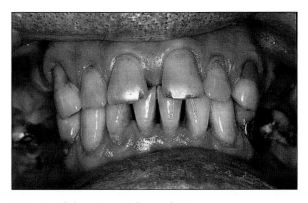

230 Good dentition. Male aged 67 years.

For the mandible, a description of a case where the connector is a lingual bar is a good starting point (**231**).

A lingual bar is made normally of cast cobalt–chromium alloy, is 3.5 mm wide and 2.5 mm thick and usually pear-shaped in section. These dimensions will ensure that the bar does not flex in function. It is generally accepted that the upper edge of the lingual bar should be at least 2.5–3 mm from the gingival margin for reasons of hygiene. A lingual bar does not provide support, indirect retention or bracing. These are obtained by prescribing rests and clasps, and placing the rests or another component anterior to the axis of rotation of the denture will produce some indirect retention. The saddles will also provide some support and bracing.

The disadvantages of the lingual bar are that it cannot have an anterior tooth added to it and, in many elderly patients, there is not enough space between the floor of the mouth and the gingival crevice to clear the bar sufficiently from the gingival crevice. The sublingual bar, which has similar dimensions but lies horizontally in the floor of the mouth rather than vertically in the sulcus has been suggested as an alternative. Although favoured by the Scandinavian countries, in our experience the anatomy of the floor of the mouth in an elderly patient, which is usually flat with no pouches sublingually (**232**), frequently precludes the use of this connector. As with the lingual bar, it is purely a connector and tooth addition is not technically practicable.

An alternative bar type connector in cobalt–chromium alloy is the dental bar (**233**, **234**). Long clinical crowns are necessary to ensure the width is sufficient to ensure rigidity without an intolerable thickness. The bar extends from below the incisal edge to 2 mm above the gingival margin. The bar has a width of 5–6 mm and a thickness of 1.2–1.4 mm. At present it is considered that the connector should span not more than six teeth.

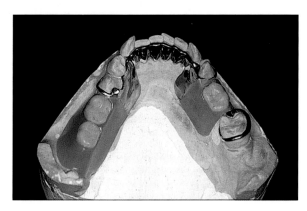

231 Lingual bar connector partial lower denture. Male aged 66 years.

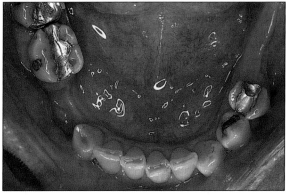

232 Typical flat shape of floor of mouth. Unsuitable for placement of sub lingual bar. Female aged 63 years.

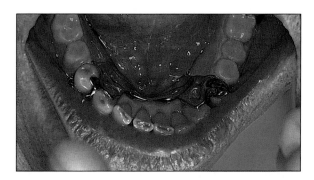

233 Try-in for partial lower denture with dental bar connector.

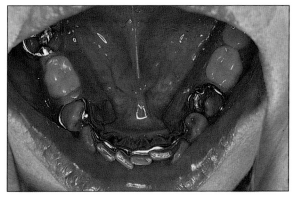

234 Partial denture (**233**) with dental bar connector in mouth. Female aged 66 years.

Where the crowns are approximately 9 mm long, it is a useful and hygienic connector. Bracing, indirect retention and some support are provided by this connector. As with the lingual bar, support and retention are also obtained through rests or clasps on suitable teeth, reinforced by saddle coverage. This connector's principal advantage, from a hygienic point of view, is that it does not cover the gingival crevice and lies above the interdental space. This is a considerable advantage where there is gingival recession associated with past periodontal disease (a not infrequent finding in the older patient).

Where there is lack of space for the lingual bar and the patient has short clinical crowns, then a lingual plate in cobalt–chromium alloy is the only alternative (**235**). To obtain maximum support, bracing and indirect retention from the lingual plate, the plate is carried almost to the incisal edges of the lower teeth. This connector, although not as hygienic as the bar connectors, is well tolerated as it is thin in section (about 0.7 mm) and less noticeable to the patient's tongue than either the lingual or dental bar. The connector is also useful and well tolerated where anterior teeth have been lost because of periodontal disease (**236–238**). When there are only a few sound teeth, the lingual plate in cobalt–chromium alloy is the connector of choice. If further anterior tooth loss occurs,

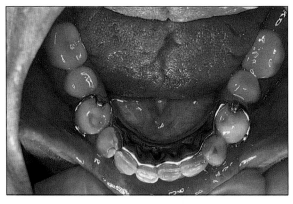

235 Lingual plate connector partial lower denture in cobalt–chromium alloy. Female aged 71 years.

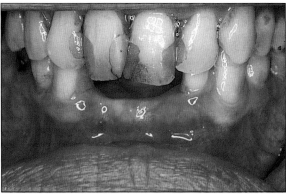

236 Anterior teeth lost owing to periodontal disease. Female aged 65 years.

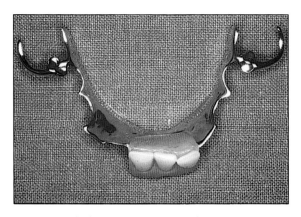

237 Lingual plate connector partial lower denture in cobalt chromium replacing 2⏐1⏐1 .

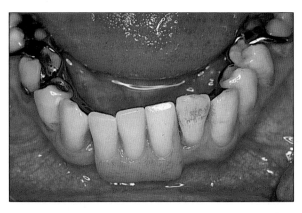

238 Partial lower denture (**237**) in place. Female aged 65 years (**236**).

addition of replacements to the plate is not technically difficult (**239**).

Patient education in cleaning the teeth and dentures and adequate recall appointments to check on dental health are always important. The lingual areas of the anterior teeth are difficult to clean so it is especially important that, when there is lingual coverage, that a regular recall is carried out to monitor oral hygiene and minimise the potentially damaging effects of tissue coverage on the lingual aspect.

In the upper jaw, the pattern of tooth loss determines the choice of connector. Where anterior teeth are being replaced an anterior palatal bar (**240**) or plate (**241**) in cobalt–chromium alloy is used. The mid-palatal bar is well tolerated by the patient if the pattern of tooth loss permits its use (**242**). Modern practice suggests that bars should cover more tissue than was originally thought. The broader coverage allows the bar to be thinner and so better tolerated. There is also the advantage that the broader coverage provides more support. Suggested dimensions are a width of 9 mm and a thickness of 0.7 mm.

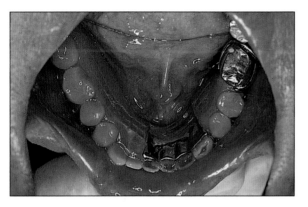

239 Lingual plate partial lower denture when only a few sound teeth remain. Male aged 72 years.

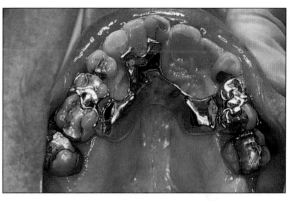

240 Anterior palatal bar partial upper denture in cobalt–chromium alloy. Male aged 72 years.

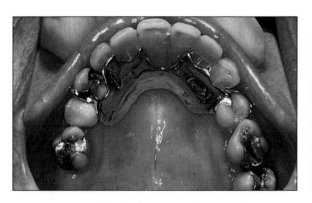

241 Anterior palatal plate partial upper denture in cobalt–chromium alloy. Female aged 72 years.

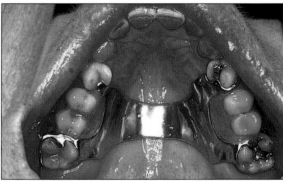

242 Middle palatal bar partial upper denture in cobalt–chromium alloy. Female aged 74 years.

The posterior palatal bar (**243**) is less commonly used. Care is necessary to ensure that the bar is correctly placed, that is, just short of the vibrating or 'Ah' line. Because of difficulties in overcoming the casting shrinkage of a long span, sometimes a small space between the bar and tissue is noticeable to the patient and this may not be acceptable. Suggested dimensions for this bar are a width of 10 mm and a thickness of 0.9 mm.

A design consisting of anterior and posterior palatal bars is still popular (**244**). The author's preference is for an anterior bar type connector in cobalt–chromium alloy. In this material, such a design is sufficiently rigid and the edentulous areas are usually large enough to allow the saddles to provide some retention, support and bracing (**245**).

When these connectors are prescribed, support and retention must be provided by suitable clasps and rests. If any of the remaining teeth are of doubtful prognosis because of a large restoration or periodontal disease, it is sensible to prescribe plate coverage on the tooth's palatal aspect. This simplifies the addition of a tooth if extraction is required at a later date.

As the number of teeth in the arch decreases it is more difficult to obtain adequate support and retention from the teeth (**246**). The bar-type connectors become a less sensible prescription and

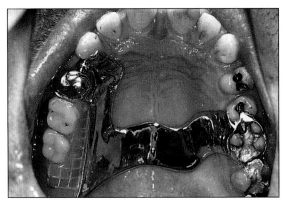

243 Posterior palatal bar partial upper denture in cobalt–chromium alloy. Male aged 59 years.

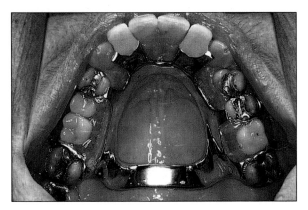

244 Anterior and posterior bar partial upper denture in cobalt–chromium alloy. Female aged 64 years.

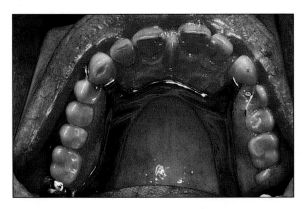

245 Anterior bar type connector partial upper denture in cobalt–chromium alloy. Male aged 67 years.

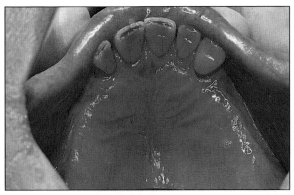

246 Large loss of teeth in upper jaw. Female aged 66 years.

consideration must be given to using palatal coverage, to obtain or supplement support and retention from the teeth (**247**). The materials used in the construction of plates are polymethyl methacrylate (**248**) or cobalt–chromium alloy (**249**). The principles of coverage are the same for both materials. The plate should extend forward from the 'Ah' line. The anterior coverage depends on the pattern of tooth loss but, where possible, the borders should be left 4 mm clear of the gingival margins; this clearance is not always possible (**247, 250**). Plates in cobalt chromium are thinner,

sharper and heavier than in acrylic. To overcome the additional weight multiple clasping is often required.

Acrylic plates are thicker and weaker but lighter and minimal clasping is often indicated in a wrought alloy. If the acrylic has a minimum thickness of 1.5 mm and adequate palatal coverage is employed, fracture during function is not usually a problem but fracture outside the mouth remains a possibility. The newer high-impact polymers may therefore offer a solution to this problem.

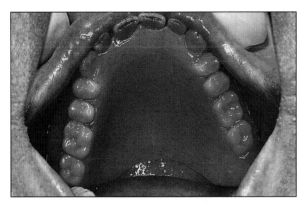

247 Acrylic plate partial upper denture with extensive tissue coverage in mouth in case shown in **246**.

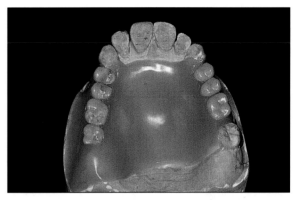

248 Wax try-in for an acrylic plate showing principles of coverage.

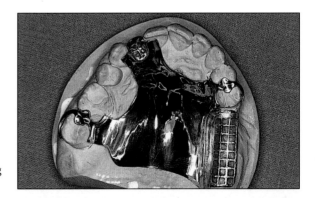

249 Cobalt–chromium alloy plate on cast showing principles of coverage.

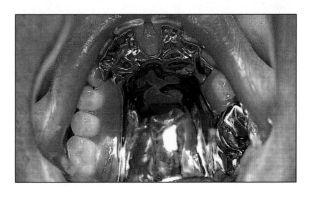

250 Almost complete tissue coverage by a cobalt–chromium alloy plate because of the pattern of tooth loss.

If fracture of an acrylic plate is a problem (**251**), then a connector in cobalt chromium is a possible solution. Because of the strength of the material, reduced coverage and weight is sometimes possible (**252**), but reduces support and retention. The provision of a partial lower denture spreads the occlusal load and reduces the risk of artificial teeth being displaced from the metal base in incision (**253**).

If the patient is conscientious about keeping their teeth, soft tissues and denture clean, and not wearing the denture at night, there seems little difference in the health of the underlying tissues whether the denture is made from cobalt–chromium alloy or polymethyl methacrylate. If oral hygiene is neglected, both materials are almost equally damaging and the condition of the remaining teeth is compromised.

The provision in the design for clasps (**254**) to provide retention, especially in the bar type of design, has been mentioned and they are often necessary when plate coverage is required. When suitable tooth undercuts are present, cast cobalt–chromium alloy clasps are effective on molar teeth as the retentive arm is long enough to be resilient in function. On premolar and canine teeth, the retentive arm in cast cobalt–chromium alloy is short because of the crown size and lacks resilience and therefore there is a risk that the clasp may break or overload the supporting tissue of the tooth. Because of this, a retentive clasp arm in wrought metal, a more resilient structure, is preferred. Wrought gold, although expensive, is the material of choice but wrought cobalt–chromium alloy or stainless steel are useful. If no tooth undercuts are present they can be made by preparing a small

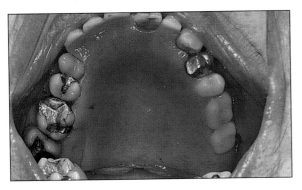

251 Acrylic plate that has repeatedly fractured. Female aged 72 years.

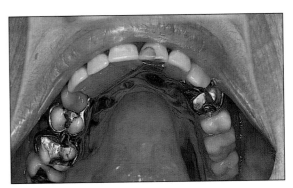

252 Cobalt–chromium alloy partial upper denture supplied as replacement for acrylic plate shown in **251**.

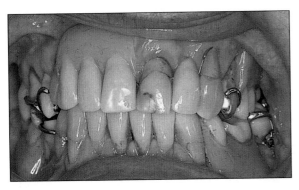

253 Cobalt–chromium alloy partial upper denture in place. A partial lower in cobalt–chromium alloy has also been supplied to spread the occlusal load (**251**, **252**). Female aged 72 years.

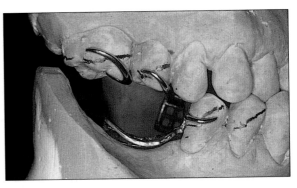

254 Occlusally approaching clasps on a cast showing the relationship of the retentive tips to the survey line.

depression in the enamel (**255**) or a restoration for a ball-ended clasp (**256**). An undercut may be produced by adding one of the composite materials (**257–259**). With recession of the gingival tissues and the risk of cervical caries, especially of the cementum, in the elderly, the preference is for occlusally rather than gingivally approaching clasps (**254**).

In partial denture design for the elderly, it is considered that precision attachments have little place as a means of securing retention and support. They are expensive for the patient and are difficult to adjust or repair. Many elderly patients find inserting and removing a conventional partial denture difficult. These problems are increased with a more complicated type of precision attachment partial

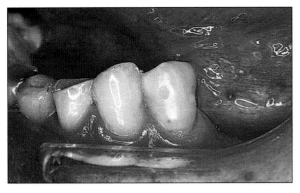

255 Small depression in enamel $\overline{5}$ prepared for engagement by a ball-end clasp.

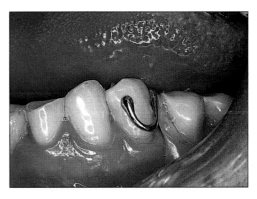

256 Ball-end clasp in cobalt–chromium alloy engaging prepared depression.

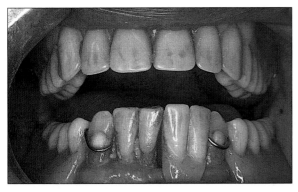

257 Artificial composite undercuts on $\overline{3|3}$ engaged by wrought clasps. Deteriorating dentition, partial lower acrylic plate. Male aged 58 years.

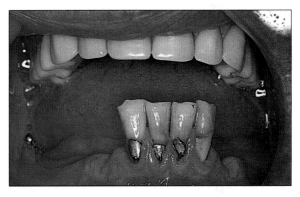

258 Recent extraction of $\overline{3|3}$. Wearing complete upper denture, with no previous experience of wearing a partial lower denture. Deteriorating dentition with $\overline{2|2}$, unsuitable shape for clasping. Male aged 74 years.

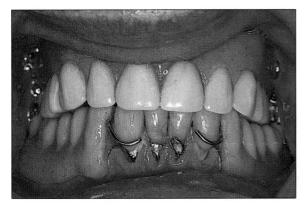

259 Composite facings on $\overline{2|2}$ providing useable undercuts to retain partial lower acrylic plate by engagement with wrought cobalt–chromium alloy clasps. (cf. **258**).

denture and, of course, it is more difficult for the patient to achieve good oral hygiene. Only for the fourth category, the difficult case because of tooth wear and problems caused by drifting and tilting of teeth, will the use of precision attachments be discussed.

The second category (**260**) has fewer teeth present, they are less sound from a periodontal viewpoint and there is the possibility of further tooth loss within a 5-year period. In many cases acrylic plates are the choice as connectors (**261**). In the upper jaw the pattern of tooth loss often requires gingival coverage (**262**). In the lower jaw (**263**), adequate tooth and soft tissue coverage is important to provide retention support and as much strength as possible. These principles are illustrated in the

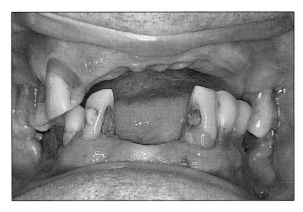

260 Patient with fewer teeth that are less sound periodontally, with the possibility of further tooth loss. Male aged 72 years.

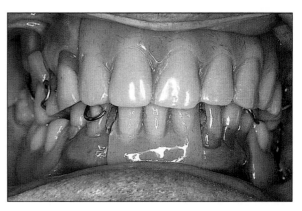

261 Case shown in **260** restored with upper and lower acrylic partial denture.

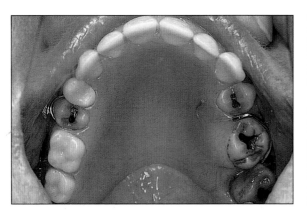

262 Complete coverage by an acrylic plate partial upper denture. Female aged 65 years.

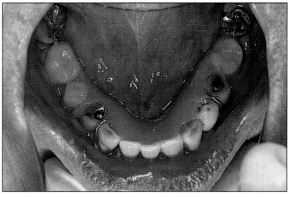

263 Acrylic plate partial lower denture. Male aged 72 years.

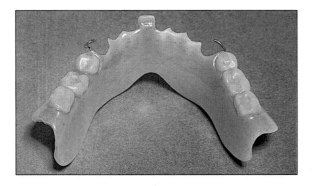

264 Lingual view of acrylic plate partial lower denture demonstrating accurate extension on to tooth surfaces and saddle areas, adequate thickness of acrylic and the use of narrow posterior teeth. These features are designed to minimise the tissue damage that can be caused by this type of denture.

view (**264**) of a partial lower acrylic plate denture. In all these cases retention and additional support are provided by clasps of wrought metal alloys. The prognosis can differ between the upper and the lower jaw. In the case in **265**, the lower dentition is likely to survive for a number of years and a cobalt–chromium alloy lingual plate (**266**) is prescribed. A history of fracture of an acrylic plate or poor toleration because of the apparent bulk of palatal coverage by acrylic can indicate the provision of a cobalt chromium plate (**267**).

Additions to the denture in acrylic or metal can be made, if there is further tooth loss, by recording an alginate impression with the denture in place. Modifications of the technique can be made when converting a partial denture to a complete

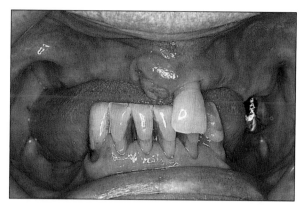

265 A lower dentition with a better prognosis than the upper dentition. Female aged 76 years.

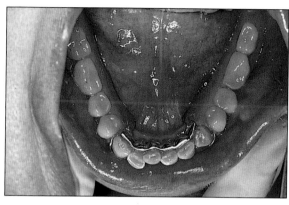

266 Cobalt–chromium alloy lingual plate supplied to the case shown in **265**.

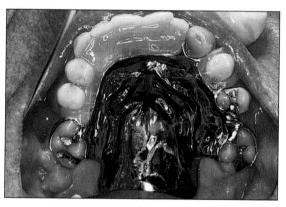

267 Cobalt–chromium alloy plate upper partial denture supplied because of poor toleration of the apparent bulk of previous acrylic denture. Male aged 69 years.

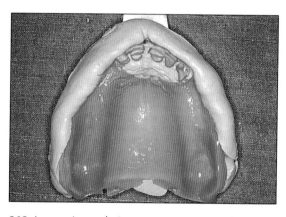

268 Impression technique to convert an acrylic partial upper denture to a complete immediate upper denture.

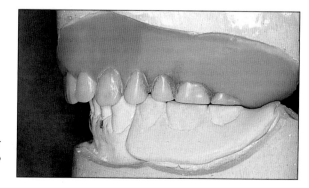

269 Cast from impression (cf. **268**) modified and anterior teeth and wax flange added prior to conversion to complete immediate upper denture.

immediate denture (**268, 269**). Dental putty can also be used as an impression material, and here an occlusal record can be made at the same time (**270**). Recent advances in denture materials that bond to metal have simplified the addition of a tooth. The bond is most effective where there is a reasonable area of metal available for bonding. If the lost tooth abuts onto the acrylic of the saddle it is always possible to add without recourse to a bonding material (**271**).

The third category is the deteriorating dentition, where some of the teeth are so diseased that the treatment planned involves extractions (**272, 273**). In most cases immediate partial dentures are indicated. These dentures are always made in acrylic with wrought clasping and are of plate design (**274**). This simple type of design is easily adjusted and allows the clinician to fulfil the promise of 'teeth out and denture in and no one will know'.

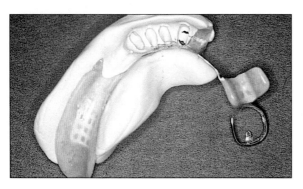

270 Dental putty impression of lower partial denture and associated oral tissue for addition of ‾3|‾ .

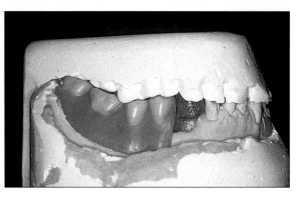

271 Cast and occlusal index from dental putty impression (cf. **270**) ready for technician to add ‾3|‾ .

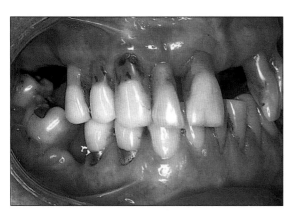

272 Deteriorating dentition. No previous denture experience 21|2 very loose. Male aged 67 years.

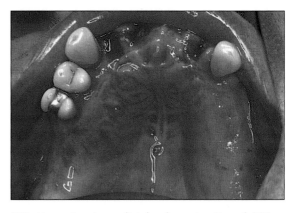

273 Upper jaw immediately after extraction of 21|2 .

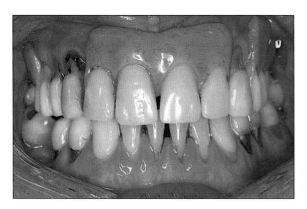

274 Partial upper acrylic plate immediate denture replacing 21|2 in place (cf. **272** and **273**).

Part or full flanges are preferable to the open-face design. Bone resorption and loss of fit can be dealt with by rebasing using one of the intra-oral rebase materials or a tissue conditioner. In some cases, immediate dentures are not indicated as the preferred line of treatment. Reasons include the wishes of the patient (**275**) or a medical condition. When initial healing has taken place (**276**) acrylic dentures of plate design with wrought wire clasping are provided (**277**). The patient's toleration of dentures can be assessed, and modifications introduced following further healing and bone remodelling.

In both these situations, the immediate denture case and the post-extraction case, replacement dentures are usually necessary when the more active phase of resorption is complete. Some of the remaining teeth are often at risk so a plate design in acrylic is often indicated. If the replacement denture is kept similar in coverage and shape to that of the original, toleration is likely to be good. In some cases the lower anterior teeth remain sound and here a cobalt–chromium alloy plate may be considered. The advantage of this type of connector when few lower teeth remain has already been described (**239**).

The fourth category of dentition is where there are problems caused by a loss of tooth tissue because of wear, drifting and tilting of teeth, or uneven distribution of teeth between the upper and lower jaw with perhaps, a history of difficulties with previous conventional partial dentures. In many of these difficult cases although the dentition may be worn it is periodontally sound. Overdentures with minimal tooth preparation or overdentures placed on teeth reduced in height after root canal therapy, with or without attachments, are therefore indicated.

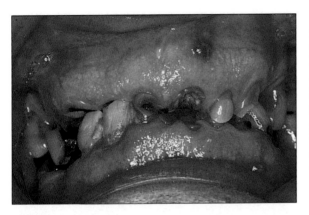

275 Neglected dentition. Patient male aged 74 years did not wish immediate dentures.

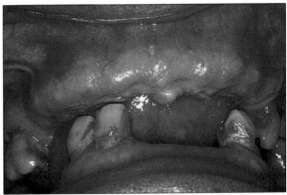

276 Initial healing complete. (cf. **275**).

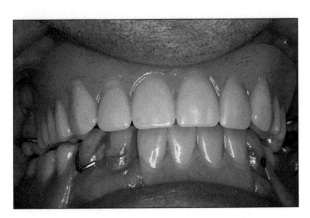

277 Restoration of function and appearance by supply of acrylic plate upper and lower dentures after initial healing (cf. **275** and **276**).

Overdentures

In the elderly patient overdentures may be prescribed in widely varying situations. This type of treatment may be appropriate where attrition has resulted in a gross loss of tooth substance on the incisal and occlusal surfaces, or where a combination of erosion and abrasion is so advanced that restoration of the labial surfaces of the anterior teeth involves the incisal edge.

The treatment of choice in a young patient, or even in the younger end of this age group, would involve the use of veneers, crowns and bridges, supplemented by partial dentures to improve posterior support, and to reduce the requirement for the periodontal ligament of the remaining teeth to oppose the occlusal load without assistance from the soft tissues (**278, 279**). Such treatment may not be feasible owing to cost, or to the patient's disinclination to submit to lengthy conservative procedures. The operator's inclination to persuade the patient to accept such a course of treatment may be tempered by the knowledge that its complexity and the risk of root caries, periodontal breakdown and longitudinal fracture of roots is likely to increase with the passage of time and that the operator's capacity to deal with these problems will be increasingly compromised by the ageing process in the patient.

Often a simpler solution will be sought and one which avoids or at least minimises further loss of tooth tissue as a prelude to restoring the dentition may commend itself to both operator and patient. In cases such as the one illustrated in **280** and **281**, very little tooth preparation would be required. It might be of assistance to round off enamel edges and to simplify the palatal surfaces. This will help to ensure that the overdenture can be fitted easily and accurately. It can be done solely by grinding or, in more advanced cases of attrition with a combination of grinding and simple restorations using glass alkenoate cements.

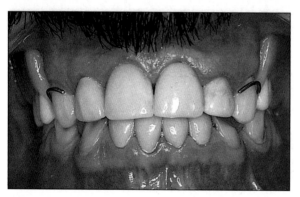

278 A combination of crown and partial denture restoration.

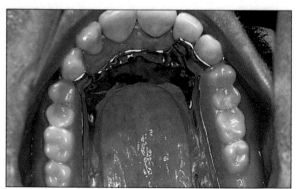

279 Palatal aspect of crowns and partial denture.

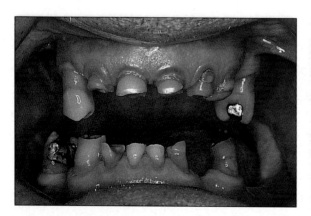

280 A case suitable for overdenture treatment.

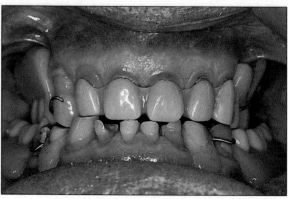

281 An overdenture alternative to crown restoration of anterior teeth.

There are a number of advantages associated with this type of prescription. The aesthetic result is usually satisfactory and the treatment process is brief. If the dentition in the opposing jaw is heavily restored, the prognosis for it will be improved because it will now be occluding evenly against a polymethyl methacrylate surface. This is undoubtedly a kinder occlusal surface than any combination of worn natural teeth, metal, ceramic or composite restorations. In such cases, the restoration of one-half of the dentition using an overdenture, with its assurance of relatively little maintenance being required, and that usually simple, may allow a more sophisticated approach in the opposing arch in the knowledge that if good posterior support has been provided, and the opposing occlusal surfaces modified as required, there are relatively few limitations on what may be attempted.

In patients displaying marked attrition, occlusal and incisal loss will still occur but it will now be concentrated in the more readily abraded polymethyl methacrylate teeth, which can be easily replaced. Where erosion and abrasion are the causative factors this may be expected to continue at the same rapid rate on any unprotected teeth but clinical observation suggests that tooth tissue protected by the overdenture will be lost much more slowly.

There are some disadvantages to overdentures. Covering gingival margins is never beneficial and covering them completely certainly incurs greater risks. The patient's assistance in maintaining oral hygiene under the prosthesis will reduce this risk to acceptable levels. Full palatal coverage will frequently be necessary, but this might be inevitable in any event with an alternative partial denture. Removal of the denture at night, which is always advised and almost always essential, may result in a dramatic loss of appearance. It should not be assumed that this will be acceptable to the patient and should be carefully discussed. This consideration should be borne in mind when upper anterior tooth reduction is being contemplated. Patients who may be prepared to accept poor aesthetics that have resulted from a slow loss of tooth substance over a long period, may be disconcerted if their appearance is suddenly modified even in a relatively minor way.

Great care must be exercised in determining how much increase in occlusal vertical dimension the patient will be able to accept. The appearance of gross loss of tooth substance may delude the operator into believing that considerable loss of occlusal vertical dimension has occurred. That this is not the case can be demonstrated by measuring the freeway space, which is almost always within normal limits, presumably owing to the continued eruption of natural teeth carrying alveolar bone with them. The safest option is to provide at least a very small freeway space when the overdenture is in place. If this still proves to be excessive, it is usually possible to reduce the vertical dimension to establish what the patient can tolerate. The anterior vertical overlap must be related to contacts in protrusion otherwise anterior teeth will be dislodged from the denture, especially if no anterior flange is being provided. Omission of the anterior flange is tempting in such cases because it improves aesthetics and reduces coverage of the gingival margins. The presence of a number of natural teeth under the denture will usually compensate for any loss of the retention associated with the provision of an anterior flange, and anteroposterior and lateral occlusal loads are unlikely to destabilise such a denture.

Overdentures with or without precision attachments may assist in the provision of partial dentures for the elderly, but care should be taken to avoid complexity.

As units of the natural dentition are lost a common problem is the large bounded upper saddle involving the anterior teeth and the premolars on one side. If opposed by natural lower teeth the patient may become quite unable to control the denture. It may fall down anteriorly because of lack of retention and be tilted down posteriorly when the patient attempts incision. Even complete palatal coverage may not provide a solution.

One answer is not to create such long saddles. Not infrequently, a tooth is added to a partial denture because it is easier and less expensive than restoring the tooth and the full implications of its loss is not appreciated by the patient or the operator until later. Such a case is illustrated in **282, 283**. A simple attachment has been used and this allows the partial upper denture to be well retained with a clasp in the fitting surface of the denture. While this is the treatment of choice,

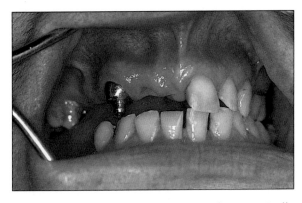

282 Retention, rather than extraction, of a strategically placed 3⌋ .

much of this advantage could have been obtained by simply retaining the root modified as described later in this chapter. Retention would be improved with the maintained ridge shape, support from the root would resist rotational forces that would otherwise dislodge the posterior part of the plate, and resorption of the edentulous saddle would be likely to be reduced since some of the masticatory load would be borne by the root. A long anterior saddle supported and retained by attachments is shown in **284**. Rapid occlusal wear, probably related to enhanced masticatory function is illustrated in **285**.

This type of device is also of use when the last good abutment tooth breaks down in a free-end saddle (**286**). Often it is difficult to justify a new crown which in any case may not be ideal for retention or support. Most of the advantage could have been gained by retaining the root under the partial denture, but further retention may be gained by using a small attachment. This will apply vertical loads to the root in a more controlled way, since the clasp will seat only when the soft tissue is slightly compressed, and lateral loads will be transmitted to

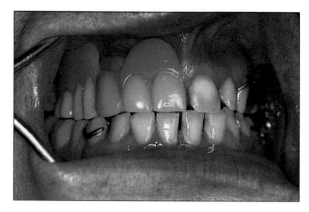

283 Overdenture restoration of the case illustrated in **282**.

the tooth at a level lower than either the tip of the tooth or the point at which a conventional clasp would apply its load. As a result, the abutment tooth would now be less likely to be compromised by movement of the denture in function (**287**).

Perhaps the most valuable contribution over-

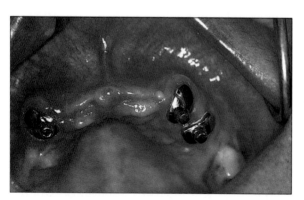

284 Retained roots with attachments to support and retain an anterior denture saddle.

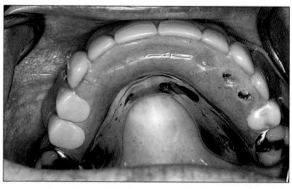

285 Rapid and extensive wear of an overdenture opposed by natural lower teeth.

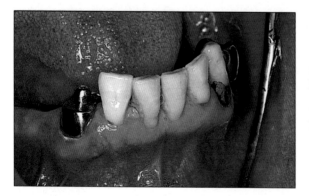

286 Retention of a former abutment tooth for an overdenture as an alternative to extraction or crowning.

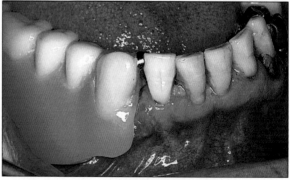

287 The restoration of the case shown in **286**.

dentures can make to the treatment of the elderly patient is at the point where consideration is being given to rendering the patient edentulous. Some time ago this might have been considered when the patient still had many or perhaps all of the anterior teeth present. Now it is more likely to occur when only two or three teeth remain in each jaw.

Retention of such teeth intact is sometimes possible (**288**), but more often it gives rise to problems. Over-eruption may disadvantageously affect both the appearance and the function of partial dentures (**289**). Fractures of such dentures may be a recurring problem. Overloading of the natural teeth may be impossible to eliminate without considerable reduction of the crowns, and this, in turn, may be impossible without devitalising the teeth. In addition, anterior natural teeth may be poorly shaped to give support to partial dentures and their distribution may lead to a loss of peripheral seal.

However, the extraction of the remaining teeth will result in occlusal loads being reduced to what can be borne by the oral mucosa without discomfort. This is usually determined by the condition of the residual ridge in the lower jaw. A pattern of ridge resorption commences which will result in the ridges becoming less and less appropriate to support, retain and brace complete dentures. At the same time the patient's purposeful muscular activity is becoming less competent to deal with the problems this causes.

Much of this can be avoided, or at least postponed by retaining the roots of some remnants of the natural dentition under otherwise complete dentures (**290**). This type of treatment may be transitional to allow the patient to accommodate gradually to wearing complete dentures or of longer duration where the roots are well positioned, periodontally sound, where the caries rate is low and the patient well motivated. It may also be appropriate where some extractions are inevitable. The presence of retained roots under immediate dentures will both assist in supporting the denture during the healing period and help to ensure optimum ridge formation in the extraction sites.

The roots of choice are canines (**291**). They are well positioned to resist incisal loads, and less likely

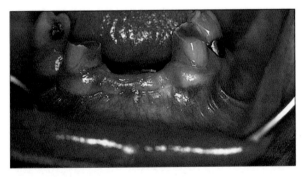

288 Residual natural teeth which create problems for conventional partial denture design.

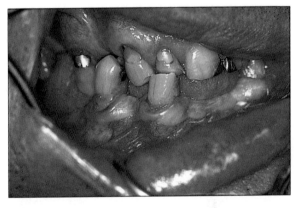

289 A combination of tooth wear and over-eruption preventing satisfactory restoration.

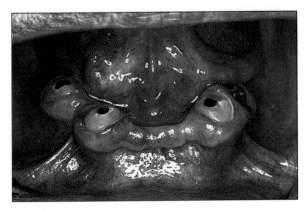

290 Root-filled decoronated lower teeth available to support and provide some retention for a complete lower denture.

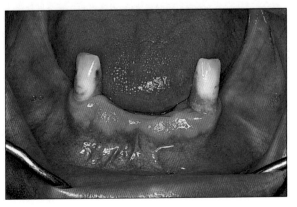

291 Lower canines suitable for overdenture treatment.

than posterior teeth to be affected by caries. They have a large root area and a simple root structure. In the lower jaw especially, additional roots in the premolar and molar regions are worth preserving, and the root of any tooth previously root filled has the added attraction that it can be retained with a minimum of inconvenience to the patient.

Patients, and especially older patients, experience greater problems with complete dentures in the lower jaw, so root retention is more important there than in the upper jaw. One root on either side of the arch is the minimum required (**292**), four widely dispersed is ideal.

The steps in carrying out treatment are reasonably straightforward. Endodontic treatment will usually, but not always, be necessary and should be carried out first. Where problems arise crowns should be sacrificed to facilitate root treatment.

Crowns should be reduced to a domed shape 1–2 mm above the gingival crevice (**293**). If possible this should be done before recording working impressions. Prior to finishing the denture the root face should be spaced from the denture with a gauge of tin foil related to the compressibility of the soft tissues. This will ensure that the roots are not loaded until the soft tissue is lightly compressed.

It is possible to reduce the crowns at the insertion of the dentures and sometimes this is the only course acceptable to the patient. If so, the operator should reduce the teeth on the cast and this reduction should be less than what is planned in the mouth. This will make denture insertion easier and

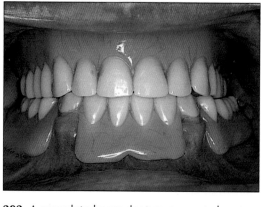

292 A complete lower denture supported on two canine roots.

the small spaces remaining can be filled with a self-curing resin. An effect similar to tin-foiling the root face can be obtained by maintaining a functional load on the denture while the resin is setting.

In many cases the retention of a small number of roots with glass ionomer restorations on the root face will achieve most of the advantages associated with more complex overdentures with attachments. Resorption will be delayed in the areas where the roots have been retained and the result will be a ridge that is often positively retentive. The height of the root dome 1–2 mm above the ridge will improve even further the capacity to resist lateral movements during masticatory function. Such a case, after 10 years, is shown in **294**.

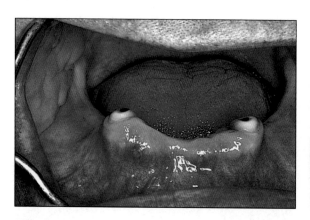

293 Canine root surface preparation following endodontics.

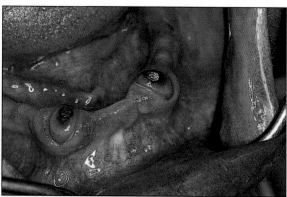

294 Some patients can maintain condition of overdenture abutments – in this case for 10 years.

Having a denture that is partly supported by natural teeth will allow the patient to apply greater occlusal loads and such patients often display the more marked occlusal wear that is normally found in edentulous patients. Recent evidence suggests that the reduction in size and density of some muscles of mastication, associated with becoming edentulous, may be postponed when overdenture techniques are employed.

Since information is still available via the receptors in the periodontal ligament, and not confined to those from the oral mucosa, which give less precise information, the patient is more aware of what is occurring at the occlusal surfaces and has better oral discrimination.

When an overdenture is supplied in the lower jaw, it is not uncommon for the patient to complain that the full denture opposing it is not well retained, so every effort must be made to maximise the forces of retention in any opposing denture, because these are likely to be fully tested. Similarly, any defect in articulation may well give rise to adverse comment.

Although not very much is being retained, patients can often be encouraged to believe that they have not yet lost all of their natural dentition and this may give some comfort.

It is only relatively seldom that complete overdentures with precision attachments would be prescribed in this age group. In cases where the ridges are very heavily resorbed, and where retention is going to be a major problem, consideration should be given to retaining canines or premolars and fitting post-retained attachments. A reasonable length of root is necessary because, on removal, the denture will apply a load in an occlusal direction and this may dislodge the post. Lateral loads applied to the root are at a slightly higher level than with simple retained roots, but this may be compensated for by the fact that application of the loads can be more finely controlled.

Where two good canines are available consideration may be given to fitting a bar between the roots. This gives the best prognosis for retaining roots because they splint each other and it is not unknown for such bars to give service for periods up to 20 years (**295–298**). Unfortunately, it is common to find that the patients with the most desperate requirement for improved retention have

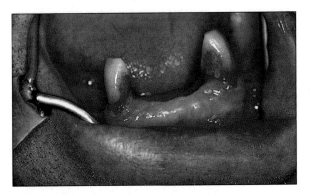

295 Treatment with a Dolder bar – initial state.

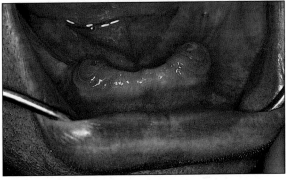

296 Tooth preparation completed.

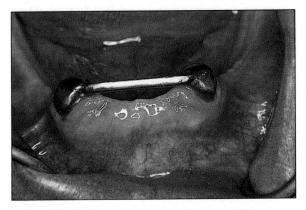

297 Dolder bar *in situ* in patient shown in **295** and **296** after 20 years.

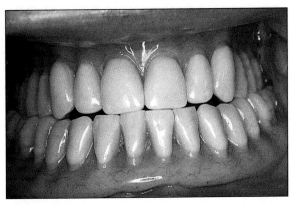

298 Complete denture in place over Dolder bar shown in **297**.

no suitable roots to provide it. By the time patients in this age group have lost most of their natural dentition anything remaining is unlikely to be suitable for precision attachments.

Further reading

Basker, R.M., Harrison, A., Ralph, J.P. & Watson, C.J. 1993. *Overdentures in General Dental Practice*, 3rd edn. British Dental Association, London.

Davenport, J.C., Basker, R.M., Heath, J.R. & Ralph, J.P. 1988. *A Colour Atlas of Removable Partial Dentures*. Wolfe Medical Publications Ltd., London.

Preiskel, H.W. 1985. *Precision Attachments in Prosthodontics, Volume II*. Quintessence Publishing Co., Chicago.

11. Complete Dentures

The aim of this chapter is to present an assessment of the requirements of the elderly edentulous population and to identify special considerations needed in helping to maintain adequate oral function. In important respects, approaches to treatment, and treatment methods themselves, require modification in order to best provide an acceptable service to an ageing population in which there are not only more old people, but also many more in the oldest age groups.

The present situation and predictions

In many countries, very large numbers of the elderly are edentulous, having grown up in environments where preservation of the natural dentition was not a high priority, in times of political and social upheaval, and before the advent of relatively recent restorative methods. In every society there exists a range of variation, and there have always been elderly individuals with sound, functional, and occasionally intact, dentitions. It is predicted that there will be a progressive shift towards long-term tooth retention as future generations reach old age. The process is already taking place and is to be welcomed. Complete dentures are a poor substitute for the natural dentition, even with the modern diet. Eventually, if current trends continue, total tooth loss may become unusual. However, the rate of change depends on the passing of generations and, in most societies, there remain large numbers of people in middle age whose dentitions have been badly damaged by caries and periodontal disease. A proportion of these dentitions will be lost, as the priority given to dental health care diminishes with age.

Irrespective of the stage at which the dentition is lost, a requirement of the dental profession is to maintain the best possible function. This requires, in turn, that the remaining oral tissues remain healthy and that the patient is provided with dentures that are as effective as possible in all aspects of function – comfort, appearance, mastication and speech – in both the short and longer term.

Health and integrity of oral structures

Earlier chapters have reviewed current knowledge of the effects of ageing and of disease processes on oral structures. In the edentulous patient, the latter have culminated in total tooth loss, but maintenance of remaining structures is required to facilitate function with complete dentures and, importantly, must be achieved despite them.

Alveolar bone loss

Rapid alveolar bone resorption follows tooth loss, even when advanced periodontal disease has been contributory to the loss. After an initial period of about a year, the rate of resorption reduces, perhaps because so-called basal bone is more resistant. It is generally considered that the presence of dentures accelerates resorption, especially in the mandible, as a result of the pressures applied during function.

As a result it is important to distribute the loading as widely as possible (**299**), and to attempt to reduce its magnitude as far as possible.

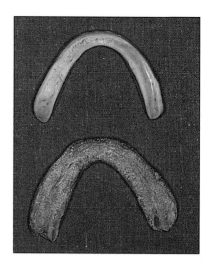

299 An under-extended lower denture, compared with a correctly extended replacement.

Mucous membrane health

The soft tissues upon which dentures are placed are at risk. Not only is the tissue subject to the presence of the dentures, but also to the age-associated changes described elsewhere. In the older patient, the risk of damage is thus greater. Localised trauma, producing ulceration in areas of high pressure is a familiar problem. More generalised damage can be a consequence of the unnecessarily high loading associated with dentures constructed to provide an excessive occlusal vertical dimension (especially if the resting vertical dimension is exceeded, and the freeway space obliterated).

Less severe local irritation maintained over a long period through lack of attention, can result in tissue overgrowth; a so-called denture granuloma is formed (**300, 301**). Typically this is infected, inflamed and oedematous and, although uncomfortable rather than painful, requires removal of the irritant feature of the denture to initiate healing.

A further form of chronic irritation of the mucous membrane under a denture is denture-induced stomatitis (sometimes called denture sore mouth, despite the absence of pain or discomfort) (**302**). Most often found in the palate under a complete upper denture, this condition has been shown in surveys of older patients to be very common. The contributory factors are: (1) continuous (24 hour) use of the denture; (2) poor or non-existent oral and denture hygiene; (3) inadequacies in adaptation of the denture to the tissues; (4) mobility of the supporting tissues and (5) occlusal errors. The red, inflamed tissue results from the presence of bacteria and yeasts in the relatively closed environment between denture and tissues. The organisms frequently adhere to the denture surface. Initial treatment should be aimed at one or more of the above factors. Medical conditions may increase the susceptibility of the tissues, as can abnormalities of the

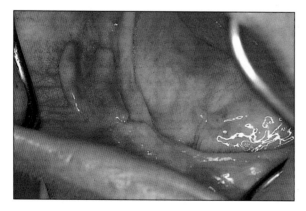

300 A denture granuloma caused by chronic irritation of an over-extended denture border.

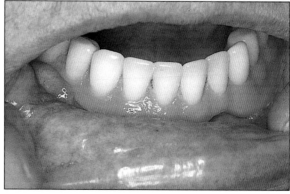

301 The denture granuloma with the offending denture in place.

mucous membrane. Such conditions may be suspected if local treatment is unsuccessful, when additional investigations may be necessary (see Chapter 13). A broad spectrum antibacterial/antifungal agent may accelerate healing in more severe cases.

Angular cheilitis is commonly associated with denture-induced stomatitis (**303**). Similar organisms may be responsible, although the lip morphology may predispose, especially in older patients in whom changes in tissue elasticity produce deep folds at the corners of the mouth.

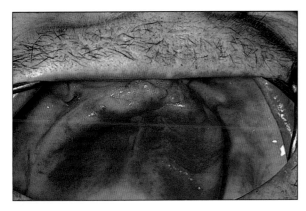

302 Denture-induced stomatitis.

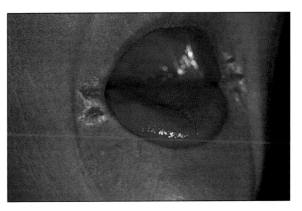

303 Angular cheilitis.

Salivary gland function

Function of salivary glands in older people has been reviewed earlier (see Chapter 4). Maintenance of a salivary film is essential for successful use of complete dentures; where there is a diminished secretion, discomfort and poor denture retention can be expected, together with mucous membrane irritation. The most common cause is xerostomia induced by drugs administered for medical reasons (see Chapters 4 and 13).

Muscle and joint function

Muscle and joint function may deteriorate. The effect of ageing upon some jaw muscles is well documented and may diminish functional capacity and precision of movement. In addition, muscle bulk and contractile properties deteriorate more in the edentulous patient than in the dentate, probably as a consequence of diminished activity even with effective complete dentures (see Chapter 4).

Temporomandibular dysfunction is observed in edentulous patients. It was previously attributed to mandibular overclosure, but is now considered either to be a consequence of a sudden change in dental occlusion, or to muscle hyperactivity caused by emotional stress. In both cases, muscle or associated connective tissue suffers temporary damage from unaccustomed loading and a period of rest is required for recovery.

Assessment of oral state

An essential feature of management of the denture-wearing patient is regular review. Since the older person is more susceptible to soft tissue damage, such reviews are of particular importance. Many of the conditions that may arise, whether of local or systemic origin, are of an insidious nature, may be unnoticed by the patient for long periods and are more difficult to manage when long-standing. A particularly serious aspect of the review process is examination for evidence of malignant or premalignant change. Early diagnosis of both is of paramount importance.

Denture maintenance

Dentures require continued care. A part of this must be provided on a day-by-day basis by the patient or the carer, whereas other aspects require attention by the dental profession.

Patient self-care

Oral hygiene is important, in order to minimise soft tissue damage (**304**). The patient, or carer, must remove the dentures for cleaning at regular intervals. Most important is avoidance of day and night wear without relief or cleaning. An ideal regime is for the dentures to be removed at night; following cleaning, most simply with soap and a denture brush, they are placed in water overnight. Dilute hypochlorite solution may be used instead of water to inhibit bacterial and yeast retention. Other cleaning agents, including proprietary products, are acceptable, but home care should avoid: (1) water temperatures above about 50°C (which damage the denture surface: **305, 306**); and (2) use of abrasive materials (toothpastes harmless to natural teeth are not suitable for dentures; **307**).

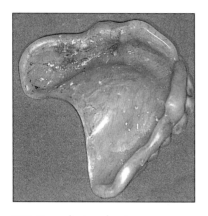

304 Poor denture hygiene.

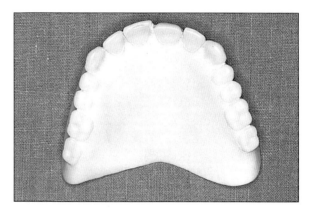

305 Opaque white denture affected by cleaning in very hot water.

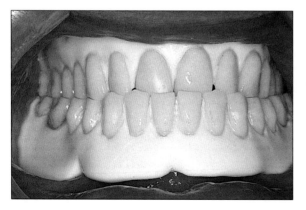

306 Appearance suffers as opacity increases. In this case boiling water had been used, after making tea at bedtime.

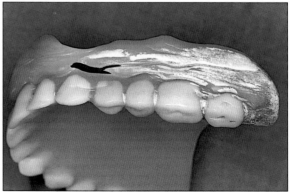

307 Abrasive damage from prolonged use of a toothpaste.

Professional care

Progressive oral changes, such as alveolar bone resorption and general deterioration of the dentures necessitate periodic action by the clinician. The oral and denture changes are commonly very gradual, to the extent that either the patient fails to perceive a decline in function or, because of the slow nature of the alteration, increasing and changing muscle skill in controlling the dentures compensates, at least until the deficiency is severe. It is important, therefore, that complete denture wearers are made aware of the need for periodic dental examination. In addition, the conscientious dental practitioner will arrange a recall system.

It is not possible to define an ideal standard recall interval. A preferable strategy is to adjust the interval between examinations to suit the patient's circumstances, with recalls ranging between 3 months and 2 years. Reasons for frequent assessment include recent extractions, past history of oral infections and medical conditions likely to affect the mouth.

At recall visits, examination will include the health of the mouth, which has already been discussed, and the state of the dentures.

Rectification of denture faults

Denture faults and deficiencies may arise from changes in the mouth over a period of time, or as a consequence of deterioration of the dentures themselves. Ultimately, it will be necessary to provide replacements, but some minor defects are best dealt with by carrying out modifications. Denture defects which may be identified at an examination fall into four general categories: (1) loss of adaptation of denture bases; (2) developing occlusal deficiency; (3) need for design change in response to change in soft tissue form and function; and (4) loss of integrity of the denture structure.

(1) Loss of adaptation

Alveolar bone resorption, and soft tissue change, diminish the accuracy of adaptation of the denture base, resulting in some loss of retention, localised trauma and discomfort (**308**). Provided that other features of the dentures are acceptable, rebasing provides an appropriate remedy. The procedure must be carried out carefully, however, otherwise the results may be disappointing and, indeed, can worsen the situation if errors occur. The objectives are to improve adaptation and border extension, without disturbance of occlusion or vertical dimension.

Clinical and laboratory details can be obtained elsewhere. However, some important points are: the need to test for and correct minor occlusal errors; an inspection for, and rectification of, under-or over-extension of the denture base prior to recording of impressions; the requirement to remove any undercut zones of the existing denture base before taking impressions. The impression material currently favoured is low-viscosity silicone elastomer, used with an adhesive. This is less likely to produce a thick overall impression layer (and displacement of the occlusion), is less irritant to the patient, and is cleaner and easier to handle, subsequently, in the laboratory. A further practical point of value is that the clinician should test the occlusion when the denture being rebased, has been seated in the mouth with the impression material, but before the latter has polymerised. The test is simple: the patient should close into normal occlusion to exclude the possibility of displacement and presence of an uneven impression film.

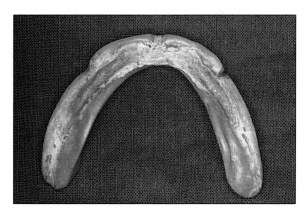

308 An ill-fitting lower denture. In this case calculus compensates for some of the loss of adaptation

(2) Acquired occlusal errors

Defects detected in denture occlusion are less readily remedied. Minor problems arising from asymmetrical function, for instance, may be overcome by occlusal adjustment. More extensive errors, and advanced overall wear (**309**) create a problem through loss of vertical dimension. Although correction is possible by addition of acrylic resin to occlusal surfaces, this is at best a temporary solution. As with rebasing, there is a risk of detracting from function rather than achieving an improvement. In general, therefore, significant occlusal deterioration is an indicator of the need for replacement dentures.

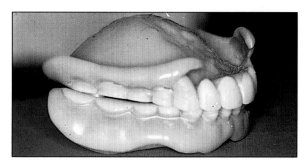

309 Advanced occlusal wear.

(3) The need for alteration to denture design

Changes in alveolar ridge form and of muscle forces applied to a denture sometimes render a hitherto successful denture unsatisfactory. An example is the loss of alveolar ridge height in the region of the mentalis muscle. A complete lower denture destabilised by the mentalis muscle, where previously it was braced by the ridge form, is unlikely to be improved by rebasing. Some polished surface recontouring may help, but there is a better case for redesigning the denture shape in the process of provision of a replacement.

(4) Loss of integrity of denture structure

It is evident that some structural defects are readily remedied. Detached teeth and localised fracture while cleaning are examples. More serious deterioration such as the surface opacity that results from exposure to hot water and abrasive damage in functional use or in cleaning require provision of replacements (**310**).

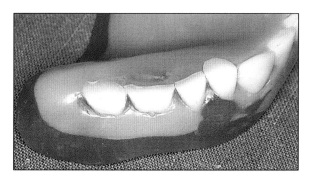

310 Advanced occlusal wear and an earlier rebase (in self-cure resin, now discoloured) render this upper denture unsuitable for further modification for continued use.

Replacement dentures

Use of complete dentures is accompanied by the generation of skills in their control, particularly during speech and chewing. Patients differ in the level of skill attained, and the rate at which it is developed. The importance of this learned muscle skill is emphasised in particular instances where dentures that are totally inadequate, as judged by normal criteria, are found in use without complaint by the patient (**311, 312**)

The widely accepted view is that such adaptation to function with dentures takes place slowly, and that it is more readily achieved by younger patients. Furthermore, once attained it is readily lost, especially in older patients if, for instance, the dentures are mislaid even for a short period.

Although the dentist can do much to facilitate the development of this skill by provision of initial dentures requiring the minimum of control by lip, cheek and tongue musculature, it is clearly of benefit to the established denture wearer if existing experience and ability can be maintained. Continued use of familiar dentures is an objective, but is subject to limits

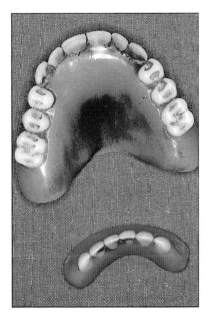

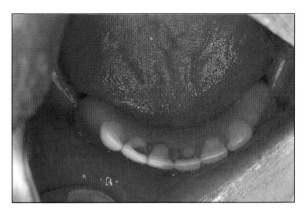

312 The fragment (**311**) was well controlled during normal speech, and was reported to be helpful during eating.

311 An elderly patient was found to be wearing a fragment of a lower denture.

imposed by tooth wear and general denture deterioration, even if successful rebasing takes place. For this reason, it has proved of great value to adopt techniques for provision of replacement complete dentures that enable selected features of existing appliances to be reproduced in the new (**313**). This approach is especially valuable, if not essential, for successful treatment of very old or frail patients.

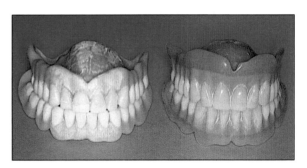

313 When provided with the new dentures shown on the right, the patient was unable to cope. The rebase already carried out may have made matters worse by increasing the vertical dimension still further.

'Copy' dentures

Regular review of the edentulous patient and assessment of dentures in use has already been advocated. The strategy provides the opportunity to select a time for provision of replacements, before deterioration and wear have become advanced. Several techniques have been described which enable the dentist and technician to copy the shapes of the old dentures, while at the same time permitting minor occlusal correction to reverse the effects of wear and allow improvement of tissue adaptation and base extension. Performed accurately, the methods require very little adaptation by the patient and are thus very effective for treatment of the older person, for whom it is especially valuable to provide an 'instant' improvement.

Full details of the technique have been published elsewhere (Davenport and Heath, 1983; Murray and Wolland, 1986); essentially, a preliminary copy of the old appliance is formed, usually from a two-part alginate mould of the denture (**314**). The mould is

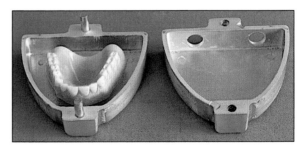

314 Metal flask to record two-part alginate mould.

filled with self-curing resin (**315**) or a combination of wax (for the teeth) and resin (**316**). The copy is then used as an impression tray and to record the jaw relationship, with correction of occlusal vertical dimension if necessary.

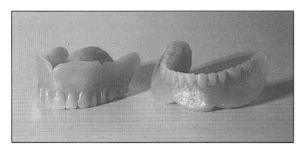

315 Poured self-cure methyl methacrylate copies, to be used to record occlusion and working impressions.

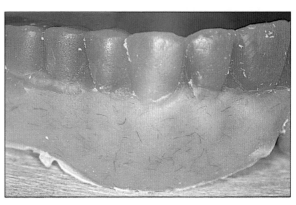

316 Detail of a copy where wax teeth are poured first, followed by an acrylic resin base.

Disadvantages of the copy technique

Clinically, simple copying of the old to formulate the new imposes limitations. If the old dentures exhibit serious defects, perhaps through extended use, it would be preferable to be able to eliminate these, while avoiding complete redesign. The acrylic resin component of the initial copy inhibits alteration, even when wax is used for tooth reproduction.

There are also some technical problems associated with the copy techniques described. In order to reproduce accurately the old denture shapes the method calls for the laboratory to remove the resin or wax teeth from the copy, ideally one at a time, and to replace each with a new denture tooth to produce a trial denture. Wax reproduction of the teeth helps, but still leaves much grinding of either tooth or base to achieve accurate setting up (**317**). This makes the technique expensive (and inappropriate for the less affluent elderly) or encourages laboratory short cuts with loss of precision.

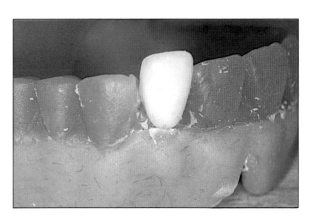

317 The potential difficulty of setting up even on a wax tooth copy is shown. A wax tooth has been removed, but either base or tooth must be extensively ground to place the new denture tooth accurately.

The replica record block technique

Although bearing a general similarity to copy techniques, and still providing the ability to copy where desired, the replica record block technique is designed to provide the clinician with record blocks derived from the original denture shapes, but which are then suitable for any modification judged desirable (Yemm, 1991). The replicas are constructed of normal dental wax, as used for conventional wax rims, but have thin rigid shellac baseplates to eliminate flexing, and to act as impression trays (**318**).

The method is applicable to any case where there are existing dentures. Alteration of the replica is as convenient as of a wax rim and involves: (1) deciding what modifications are needed to improve the shape and form of new dentures; and (2) addition and removal of wax from each record block to achieve the objectives. The fundamental difference between this approach, and the use of conventional wax rims is that the new prescription can be orientated towards the individual patient, rather than depending upon the operator's perception of the requirements. Only intended changes are introduced into the prescription. For instance, modification of one denture may be needed, while the other can be reproduced virtually unaltered. The prescription to the laboratory is precise and the process of setting up is not inhibited by the presence of acrylic resin.

The method has been in use for some 10 years and has proved successful in general dental practice and in the dental laboratory. Clinical success rates, especially with older patients, are higher than with conventional methods, as judged by the frequency with which patients are immediately able to report improved comfort and function, rather than experiencing a protracted period of limited success.

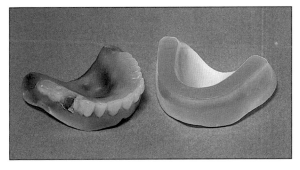

318 An upper replica record block compared with a conventional wax rim constructed for the same patient. Although both are readily modified, the replica provides a more appropriate starting point.

Clinical and laboratory stages, replica record block technique

The wider application of this method, compared with techniques reserved for circumstances where copying is appropriate, warrants a brief description of clinical and laboratory procedures.

Stage 1 (Clinic)

The patient and existing dentures are examined carefully. In addition to normal inspection of the mouth, a list of defects in the dentures is developed, and plans for alteration devised. A simple check-list is convenient. An example is shown in **319**, devised initially for undergraduate use.

On completion of the detailed treatment plan, impressions of the existing dentures are recorded, using an inexpensive laboratory silicone putty. The dentures are not modified prior to this process,

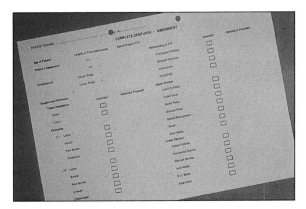

319 A check-list for treatment planning for complete dentures. The form provides for identification of faults, and a note of the correction proposed.

except where major under-extension of borders is identified. In this event, the extension is temporarily corrected using greenstick tracing compound (**320**). The impressions, which form a mould, are recorded in two parts: first the polished surface (**321**) and then the denture base (**322**). The dentures are returned immediately to the patient (**323**) after removal of any tracing compound.

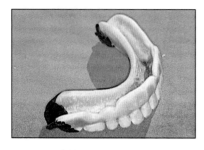

320 An old lower denture prepared by tracing-compound correction of distal under-extensions.

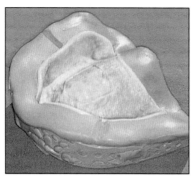

321 The first part of the silicone mould. Note the use of a plastic tray and the creation of a flat border of silicone around the denture, which is embedded up to its borders. Small locating notches have been cut to locate with the second part of the mould.

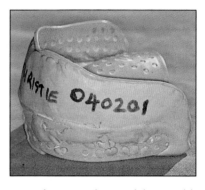

322 The second part of the mould. The second tray is used inverted. A separating medium (e.g. emulsion hand cream) is essential. Labelling is with indelible pencil.

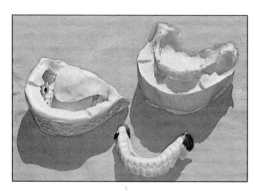

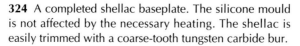

323 The mould opened. The tracing compound is removed, and the denture returned to the patient.

Stage 2 (Laboratory)

Using the two-part mould, the laboratory constructs replica record blocks. Baseplate shellac is placed on the impression of the denture base, heated and adapted. The extension of the baseplate is reduced to that of the original denture (**324**) and secured in place on the silicone with wax. Pour-ways are cut in the posterior regions, and wax poured into the residual cavity, at a temperature of approximately

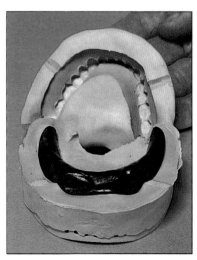

324 A completed shellac baseplate. The silicone mould is not affected by the necessary heating. The shellac is easily trimmed with a coarse-tooth tungsten carbide bur.

100°C (**325**). After cooling, the replicas are removed and require only removal of the sprues and minor tidying and polishing prior to clinical use (**326**).

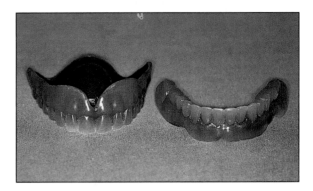

326 Completed replica record blocks after removal of sprues and polishing.

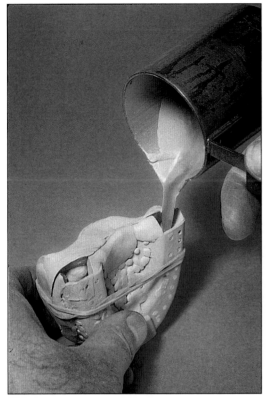

325 Pour-ways cut posteriorly and wax poured with the mould closed with a rubber band. The shellac baseplate is in place.

Stage 3 (Clinic)

On the patient's second visit, the record blocks are modified by adding and removing wax to conform with the treatment plan. Modification is not inhibited by the record block material. Examples of possible alterations include (**327–329**) changes to occlusal vertical dimension, repositioning or reorientation of

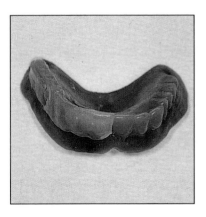
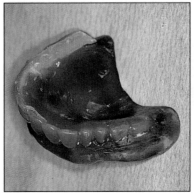
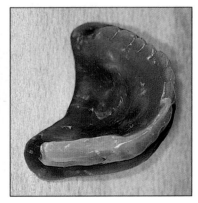

327–329 Three views of an upper replica. One side is unchanged. The other demonstrates some of the scope for alteration, including changes to the occlusal plane (add or subtract) alteration to anterior tooth position and movement of posterior teeth to change arch shape.

occlusal plane, alteration to anterior tooth position (for appearance or denture stability) and changes in posterior tooth position to improve tongue space.

At the same visit, wash impressions are recorded in the record blocks using a low-viscosity silicone elastomer, with an appropriate adhesive to secure the material to the shellac base (**330**). Condensation curing materials are preferred, since setting time can be adjusted and the adhesives are more effective. Prior to taking impressions, the border extension is adjusted. A closed-mouth impression technique is recommended, in which the patient closes into occlusion during the polymerisation process of the impression material, in one replica at a time. This method reduces the risk of introducing an occlusal error by uneven placement.

Generally, the impressions are recorded after modification of the wax rims. However, if the original dentures were very poorly adapted, the record blocks will be rendered more manageable if impressions are recorded prior to modification of the wax superstructure.

On completion of record block alteration and impressions, the jaw relationship is recorded; this is done most conveniently with a bite-recording paste (**331**). This should be arranged to adhere to one occlusal surface, and to locate (with small key-ways) on the other surface (**332**).

Finally, the teeth (shade, mould, occlusal form) and appropriate articulator are selected.

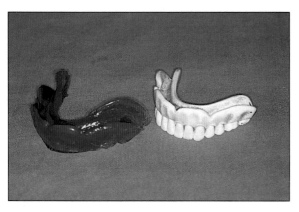

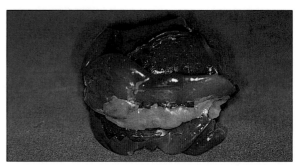

331 The jaw relationship recorded with bite-recording paste, which is employed with an adhesive on one record block only.

330 A modified lower replica with a completed impression. Comparison with the original shows improved distal and disto-lingual extension, partly defined prior to recording of the silicone mould (see **320**). It is essential to use an effective adhesive prior to impression recording.

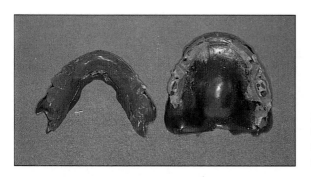

332 The record blocks separated to facilitate impression casting. Note the small locating grooves cut in the occlusal surface of the lower block to ensure accurate relocation.

Stage 4 (Laboratory)

The laboratory separates the record blocks, casts the impressions, reassembles the occlusion and mounts the casts on the articulator chosen.

The modified replicas provide an accurate prescription and the technician is readily able to comply with the detail by setting up on the replica

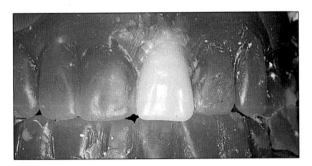

333 Setting up: in this case the original tooth position is being copied, and the example demonstrates the potential accuracy.

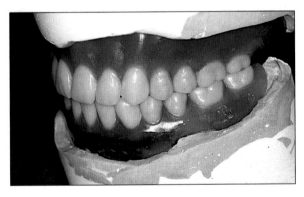

334 Completed trial dentures.

bases. Progressive removal of small sections of the wax and substitution by new denture teeth, ensures that the clinician's prescription is retained (**333**). The process is not hindered by an increased need to grind teeth.

Once setting up is completed, the wax-up process is generally simple, since the proposed polished surface shape has already been defined by the clinician. A final step is removal of the impression borders and replacement with wax to the sulcus depth recorded on the cast (**334, 335**).

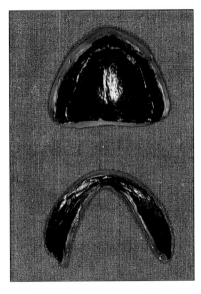

335 Trial dentures removed from the casts to demonstrate the retention of the impression material except at the borders, which have been rewaxed.

Stage 5 (Clinic)

The clinical trial stage is conventional, although notable for the reduced incidence of problems requiring rectification and retrial. This is, in part, due to the improved precision of prescription and, in part, because there is less chance of major error in recording the jaw relationship.

Stages 6 (Laboratory) and 7 (Clinic)

Laboratory completion, and subsequent clinical insertion of the finished dentures follow normal procedures. After-care should be arranged as always with new dentures.

The patient with no dentures

Most edentulous patients present with existing dentures. Even if these are very poor, the replica method is preferred, especially if the patient has used them for a long period (**336, 337**). However, accidental loss, and sometimes dental clearance without provision of immediate dentures, requires adoption of conventional techniques. These are well documented in other texts. Some general indicators may be helpful in applying standard methods to older patients.

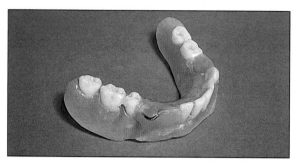

336 This partial denture had been worn successfully for many years prior to sudden loss of the remaining teeth. Wax has been added to complete the arch prior to recording the silicone putty mould.

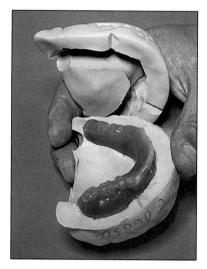

337 A replica of the denture shown in **336**.

Impression taking

Many old people dislike intensely the impression process. In part, this may be from recollection of older techniques, such as use of impression plaster. The discomfort and insecurity may be minimised by recording wash impressions in special trays constructed from preliminary alginate records, or in record blocks with rigid bases, using low-viscosity silicone (and an adhesive), and by ensuring that the patient is sitting upright.

Denture shapes

In the absence of denture-wearing skills, minimum bulk of appliances should be ensured, together with attempts to place the dentures in the neutral zone, perhaps by recording an impression of the most readily available space (**338**)

For some patients, it may be wise to provide an upper denture first, leaving construction of the lower until the patient has mastered the (easier) upper.

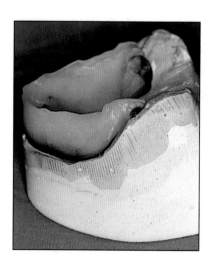

338 A neutral zone impression (piezogram). A lower denture constructed to this shape should suffer as little as possible from displacing forces.

Vertical dimension

If the patient has been accustomed to functioning without dentures (**339**), instant provision of appliances with a 'normal' freeway space of 2–4 mm will impose a major change. Even in the case of those used to dentures, but where occlusal wear is advanced, a more gradual return to normal occlusal vertical dimension may be more easily tolerated.

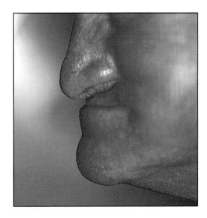

339 Habitual closure to this extent should be respected by incorporating a large free-way space into complete dentures provided.

Jaw relationship

In the absence of dentures, or where gross occlusal wear has occurred, abnormal jaw-closing pathways are often adopted (**340**). In some patients these may be abandoned rapidly once an improved occlusion is provided, but in others they may persist. A suitable compromise is to record, as far as possible, a jaw relation with the mandible retruded, but to use cuspless (zero-angle) posterior teeth, which permit variation of the closed position by avoiding a specific intercuspal relationship.

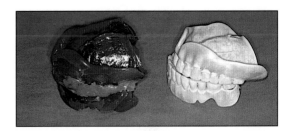

340 A comparison of a new retruded jaw position with that adopted by the patient with old dentures. The patient may not immediately use the retruded position, but use of cuspless teeth will allow freedom.

Management of damaged denture-bearing tissues

Although there are advocates of surgical modification of the mouth prior to treatment to provide new dentures, this is best restricted to the very occasional extreme case of tissue overgrowth, especially where the patient is elderly (see Chapter 14).

Tissue conditioners

A useful alternative method that allows tissue recovery is the use of so-called tissue conditioners. Applied to the denture base as a temporary lining, these are helpful in reversing the effects of trauma, partly by their elasticity and partly by possession, at least briefly, of the ability to flow (**341**).

Most tissue-conditioning materials involve gradual formation of a polymer gel in a solvent. Loss of the solvent limits the useful life of the lining in such cases.

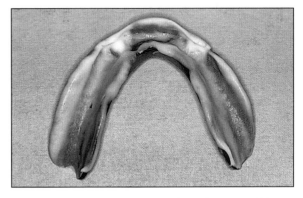

341 A tissue conditioner (Viscogel) applied to an ill-fitting lower denture.

Functional impression techniques

Variability of the thickness and physical character of soft tissue underlying complete dentures is thought to contribute to discomfort, especially in the case of the lower jaw. One widely supported approach is to employ muco-displacive impression techniques to develop the fitting surface of a new denture. This involves an attempt to simulate functional loading by means of a high-viscosity impression material, used in a fashion likely to displace mobile tissue. There are doubts about the extent to which this simulates actual functional (usually asymmetrical) loading, as the effect is to produce a denture that is closely adapted to the tissues only when under load.

An alternative method, designed to accommodate, variable tissue features, is to use a functional impression technique. This involves addition of a visco-elastic lining to an existing denture. The denture is then used in a normal fashion by the patient, during which time the material is assumed to flow to redistribute pressures. After a period of a few days the denture is retrieved from the patient and rebased. The process may be employed either as an alternative to conventional rebasing of an earlier denture (**342, 343**), or as a means of final production of a fitting surface on a new denture. The technique has its greatest application on the lower jaw. The materials are commonly similar to those used as tissue conditioners, although there are, in addition, some visco-elastic polymers available in sheet form (**344**). Overall, clinical results encourage wider use of this method, and it may reduce the need to resort to provision of a soft lining for a lower denture. Even the most recent materials for this purpose pose problems of denture hygiene and have relatively short useful lives – both problems of particular relevance in treatment of older patients.

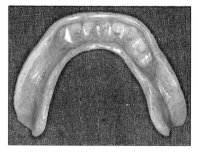

342 A complete lower immediate denture. Alveolar bone resorption has caused uneven loading and discomfort.

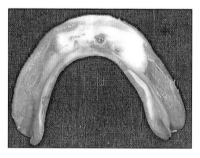

343 A functional impression recorded over several days, which will be used to rebase the denture.

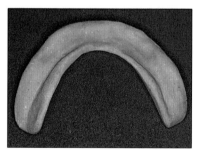

344 A functional impression recorded with a sheet-material (Ardee).

References

Davenport, J.C. & Heath, J.R. 1983. A copy denture technique. *British Dental Journal*, **155**, 162–163.

Murray, I.D. & Wolland, A.W. 1986. New dentures for old. *Dental Practice*, **24**, 106–109.

Yemm, R. 1991. Replacement complete dentures: no friends like old friends. *International Dental Journal*, **41**, 233–239.

Further reading

Basker, R.M., Davenport, J.C. & Tomlin, H.R. 1992. *Prosthetic Treatment of the Edentulous Patient*, 3rd edn. MacMillan, London.

Grant, A.A., Heath, J.R. & McCord, F. 1994. *Complete Prosthodontics: Problems, Diagnosis and Management.* Mosby–Wolfe, London.

12. Implants

The objective of this chapter is to provide a brief introduction to the use of modern implant techniques to improve the performance of prostheses. Replacement of one or a small number of missing teeth is best achieved with a fixed device, supported by adjacent natural teeth, and thus using biological support. When there has been loss of large numbers of teeth and, in particular, when the patient is edentulous in one or both jaws, the use of fixed appliances is no longer possible and a denture must rely heavily or completely upon residual structures (345, 346).

Numerous attempts have been made to devise methods to overcome the deficiencies of large or complete dentures, including transplantation of teeth from donors, implantation of metal structures between bone and periosteum (subperiosteal implants) and the insertion of structures into the bone. In the last two cases, the objective was to provide intra-oral projections on which to attach a denture and to give enhanced support of functional loading and retention. Success of these attempts has, until recently, been, at best, poor and most

have been abandoned. The common biological response has been down-growth of epithelium from the site of projection into the oral cavity, with progressive separation of the implant, looseness, infection and eventually removal is required.

Another approach, based on the assumption that a significant limiting factor on denture function was advanced alveolar bone resorption, has been to attempt to improve the form of the residual alveolar ridge, both by modification of soft tissue (sulcus deepening) and by ridge augmentation with bone, bone derivatives or inorganic analogues of bone. Some of the augmentation techniques have been abandoned and others remain experimental. In any case, even if successful, the procedures still require the patient to learn to control essentially mobile dentures.

More recently, improved materials and more careful techniques have led to the development of a form of intra-bony implant, where close approximation of implant and bone provides both rigidity of the implanted structure and inhibition of the epithelial down-growth and implant rejection.

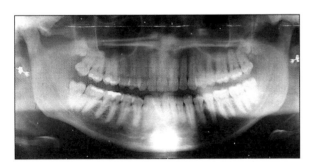

345 The natural dentition.

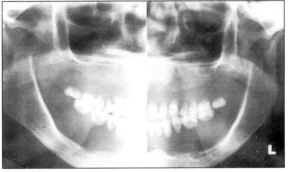

346 Complete dentures relying upon resorbed alveolar ridge structures.

Osseointegration

Osseointegration is the descriptive term applied to a process whereby a biologically inert material, implanted into bone, becomes rigidly fixed by bone deposition and is able to transmit applied loads directly from implant to bone (**347**).

The features of the process were first described by Branemark (for a review see Branemark *et al.*, 1977), together with a clinical and technical process for its application to problems in replacement of tooth loss. The original method depended on innovative implant design, construction of the implants of commercially pure titanium and extreme care to avoid contamination during implant insertion. In addition, no load was applied to the implants for a period of 4–6 months after insertion to allow bone healing (integration) to occur. In the Branemark system, this is achieved by completely covering the implants for this initial phase and adding the transmucosal superstructure at a second surgical operation.

Since the introduction of this, other implant systems have been developed. Some have simplified the surgical procedure by allowing implant projection into the mouth at the insertion, but without applying load during the integration phase. In addition, ceramic and bone constituent implants have been produced, primarily for use in the replacement of single teeth. The reader is directed to specialist publications for more detail.

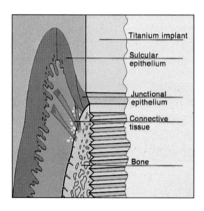

347 Diagrammatic representation of the relationship between implant and biological tissues.

Application of osseointegrated implants

The potential advantages and disadvantages of implants are summarised in **Table 46**. In general, the advantages identified are in improving functional ability with a prosthesis, while disadvantages stem from the increased complexity of initial treatment and aftercare.

In general use, the technique of implantation has proved more successful than any previous method. Multicentre studies, particularly of the Branemark system, carried out on large diverse population groups have indicated success rates for individual implants of over 85% on 10-year observation periods. Since the use of multiple implants in a single jaw is

Table 46. Treatment indications and contraindications.

Indications

1. Inability to retain comfortably and wear a removable prosthesis as a result of severe morphologic compromise of denture bearing areas, presence of hyperactive gag reflex, etc.
2. Apparent inadequacy of oro-muscular coordination (e.g. Parkinson's disease, dykinesias, etc).
3. Intolerance of prostheses supporting tissues.

Contraindications

1. Patient's systemic health is brittle or uncontrolled.
2. Proposed host bone sites demonstrate quantitative or qualitative compromise.
3. History of drug abuse.
4. Serious mental health disturbances.
5. Dentist judged unrealistic expectations regarding aesthetic results as perceived by the patient.

commonly advocated, single implant failure may still be consistent with functional success.

To date, the procedure has mainly been applied to younger patients and evidence of routine use for older patients is quite sparse, especially as regards long-term maintenance.

Some additional features of current results are:

- The anterior regions of both mandible and maxilla are most readily able to accept implants. Posteriorly, anatomical features such as the maxillary sinus and inferior dental canal present problems.

- Bone loss following successful integration seems to be less than would be expected with conventional denture wearing.
- Long-term soft tissue responses appear to be favourable, at least over the observation periods available and in the presence of appropriate self-care and professional review. The presence of plaque around an implant does not appear to have an irreversibly detrimental effect on adjacent soft tissue (**348, 349**).
- In the event of implant failure, removal is followed by rapid healing of the bone defect.

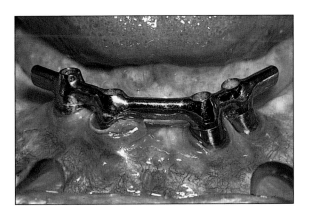

348 Tissue damage caused by lack of self-care.

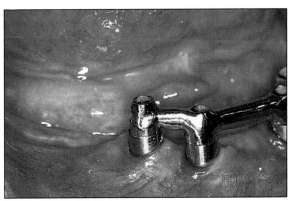

349 A return to healthy state after modification of oral hygiene regime and superstructure.

Patient selection

It is widely agreed, that patient selection is of critical importance. Treatment involves a surgical procedure to insert the implants and an extended healing period before the final superstructure can be constructed. In assessment of an older patient, it must be ascertained that the surgery and healing period can be tolerated. This inhibits the application of the technique to many frail or medically compromised people.

In addition, there is general agreement that self-care and attendance for professional review are essential for maintenance. The potential patient's motivation requires careful assessment.

Persistent problems with the results of conventional tooth replacement methods are powerful indicators for alternative treatment, especially if repeated attempts have been made to achieve an acceptable result.

Table 47 summarises indications and contra-indications.

Table 47. Use of implant techniques for elderly patients.

Advantages

Improved support and retention.
Enhanced function (chewing, speech, etc).
Greater confidence.
Reduced dependence on denture-wearing skill.

Disadvantages

Need for surgery (medical status, tolerance).
Extended treatment period before advantages accrue.
Need for continued self-care (motivation? ability?)
Need for regular professional review.
Risks of failure in very old age – loss of control skills.

Insertion of implants

Following initial selection of a patient for possible implant treatment, a careful radiographic analysis of the proposed implant sites is carried out. Included in this is the assessment of bone quantity and quality, upon which the decision on the number and length of implants depends (**350–352**). A surgical template may be fabricated for use as guide to optimal location of the implants, although discrepancies between the soft tissue ridge and underlying bone crest can detract from the value of such a template. One of the most important objectives is placement to enable transmucosal components to lie within the body of the eventual prosthesis without distortion of the required tooth position. The template is therefore best developed from a new denture constructed prior to the decision to use implant techniques, and designed to be a prototype, at least for tooth position (**353, 354**).

Pre-surgery planning also includes final decision on the eventual superstructure type (fixed or removable), which is dependent not only on patient and operator preferences, but also on implant numbers and orientation (**Table 48**).

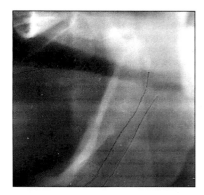

350 Radiograph of mandible.

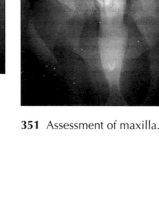

351 Assessment of maxilla.

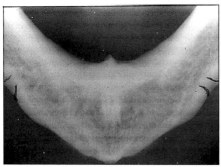

352 Position of inferior dental canal.

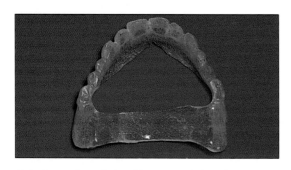

353 A template derived from an existing denture.

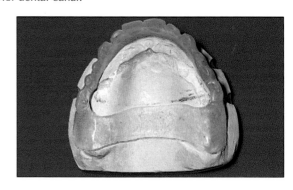

354 Template in position on cast.

Table 48. Multicentre prospective studies suggest the following considerations for decision-making regarding prosthodontic design for geriatric patients.

Arch	Number	Implants Length	Implants Orientation*	Resorption pattern**	Prosthodontic treatment	Length of cantilevers
Mx	6/5	≥10 mm	1	1 or 2	Fixed	<10 mm
Mx	4/<4	10 mm or >10 mm	1 or 2	2 or 3	Overdenture	—
Md	5	≥10 mm	1	1, 2 or 3	Fixed	<15 mm
Md	4	≥10 mm	1	1, 2 or 3	Fixed	>10 mm
Md	4	≥10 mm	2	1, 2 or 3	Overdenture	–
Md	<	≥10 mm	1 or 2	1, 2 or 3	Overdenture	–

* Implant orientation in either arch:

1.   semi-lunar;   2.   closer to a straight line.

● ● ● ●   ● ● ● ●

Mx: maxilla

Md: mandible

** Resorption of alveolar bone in either arch:

1. mild; 2. moderate; 3. severe

Insertion of implants can be performed under local or general anaesthesia. The implants themselves, and all other equipment are subject to aseptic techniques to avoid bone infection and contamination of the metal surfaces. Bone cutting is performed with great emphasis upon temperature control. The implants, which in most systems are constructed of titanium, may be threaded or plain cylinders, solid or hollow. In the Branemark system they are inserted so that the implant surface is flush with, or just below, the cortical surface of the residual ridge and then covered by the replaced mucoperiosteal flap. In other systems the aim is to leave the surface just above the replaced flap. Implant length is determined by available bone depth; an ideal outcome is for the 'apical' end of the implant to engage cortical bone (for instance, at the lower border of the mandible).

After initial recovery for a period of 8–10 days the patient can usually return to wearing a conventional denture, suitably modified and provided with a temporary soft rebase. The implants must not be loaded, and must remain so for a period of 4–6 months, during which time bone growth to produce integration is expected. Transmucosal attachments for the superstructure are then added, either at a second surgical session (Branemark), or by removal of temporary cover screws (e.g. Bonefit). After mucosal healing, where necessary, work to provide the superstructure can be initiated.

The prosthesis

The superstructure can be fixed to the implants or may be removable. A fixed appliance requires more implants and, because of the limitation of these to anterior regions, requires some degree of cantilever effect to provide some posterior occlusion. In contrast, removable appliances require fewer implants and are commonly provided with a conventional extension of the denture base, in which case, the implants provide an aid to support and retention of the appliance rather than being the sole source. The decision regarding fixed or removable appliances will have been made after careful assessment in conjunction with the surgeon, prior to implant placement.

Table 49. Problems and complications related to implants.

Time	Description
Stage I surgery	Unfavourable implant placement or alignment
Following Stage I	Swelling and ecchymosis Suture remnants Wound dehiscence
Stage II surgery	Failure to osseointegrate Inability to use implant(s) effectively Problems with abutment connection
Following prosthodontic treatment	Soft tissue complications Prosthodontic complications and maintenance considerations
Delayed complications	Late implant loss Neuropathies

Table 50. Prosthodontic complications and maintenance considerations.

Type	Description
Structural	Implant fracture* Abutment screw fracture*,† Damaged abutment screw components*,† Gold alloy screw fracture*,† Cast framework fracture* Adjustment/Repair of Retentive unit† Frequent need for relining distal extension areas†
Cosmetic	Unfavourable pontic(s) placement* Display of metallic components* Incorrect labial/buccal flange design*,†
Functional	Speech problems* Transient discomfort of muscles of mastication*,†

* Fixed and † overdenture prosthesis

The removable appliance

This may be the most appropriate use of implants in the elderly patient, in particular as an aid to solving difficulties with the complete lower denture. Only a limited number of implants is needed, thereby minimising the extent of the surgical procedure. The implants may be connected by a cast bar

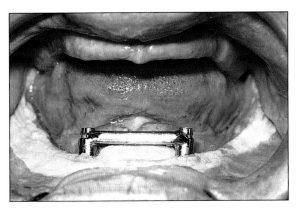

355 Bar connector.

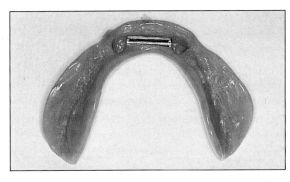

356 Complete lower denture with attachment to bar (**355**).

(**355**), and the denture attached to the bar by means of a sleeve, to provide support and retention (**356**). Alternatively, individual implants may carry attachments with corresponding components in the denture base (**357, 358**).

A similar approach is possible for the upper denture. Although it is more often possible to achieve satisfactory function by conventional means, difficult circumstances, such as a hyperactive gag reflex, may limit palatal coverage and encourage the use of an implant solution.

The process of provision of the implant-borne denture is aided by preliminary development, prior to implantation, of the best possible conventional appliance. This can then form the basis for the final denture design, perhaps employing a modification of the replica record block method (see Chapter 11).

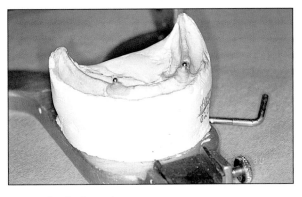

357 Individual attachments.

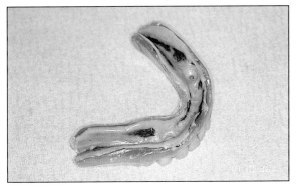

358 When completed, this lower denture will incorporate components to attach to individual retainers (**357**).

The fixed appliance

In addition to the requirement for a larger number of successfully integrated implants, the provision of a fixed appliance is more demanding not only in its construction, but also in subsequent maintenance. For several reasons, therefore, this form of treatment may be less frequently the wise choice for the older patient. A case illustrated here is that of a 'young' old person who had retained his lower dentition and had demonstrated his ability to undertake adequate self-care to control periodontal disease. Implant treatment in the edentulous upper jaw has a major advantage in prevention of progressive damage to the soft tissue and bone, which would otherwise be heavily loaded under a conventional complete upper denture opposed by natural lower teeth.

Using the Branemark system, the stages of treatment are as follows:
1. Radiographic assessment, and the decision that bone features permit surgical insertion of an

adequate number of implants to meet the prosthodontist's criteria for eventual provision of a fixed appliance (**359**).

2. After implant placement and osseointegration period, transmucosal components are added (**360**).
3. In the meantime, the patient wears a modified conventional denture (**361**).

4. After healing has been completed the mouth is ready for superstructure construction (**362**).
5. A special tray is constructed, allowing laboratory access to transfer copings to be placed on each implant (**363**).
6. Transfer copings are then placed, and united by a rigid temporary self-curing resin bridge (**364**).

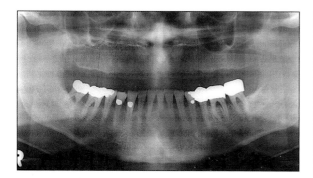

359 Radiographic assessment: natural lower dentition and maxillary bone structure.

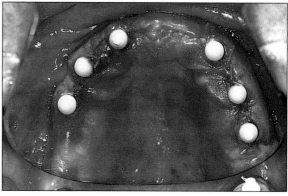

360 Implants in place with transmucosal components.

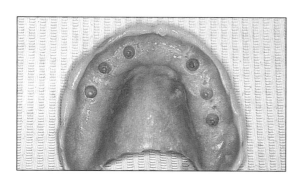

361 Modified conventional denture for temporary use.

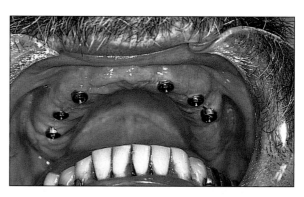

362 Healing period completed.

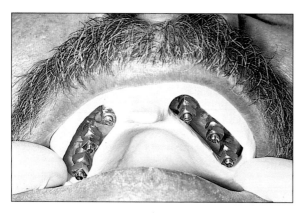

363 Special tray with access to transfer copings.

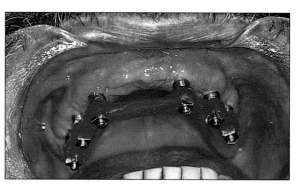

364 Transfer copings connected.

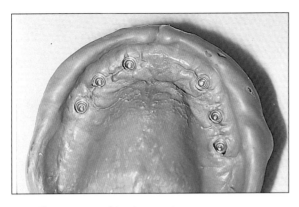

365 Elastomer working impression.

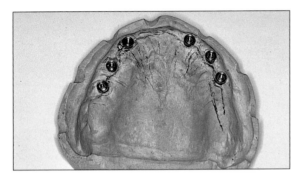

366 Cast obtained after brass analogues inserted into impression.

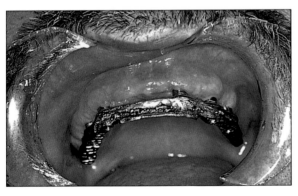

367 Trial of cast superstructure.

7. An impression is recorded using a suitable elastomer. The transfer copings are removed with the impression, their relationship maintained by the resin bridge (**365**).
8. A working cast is produced, reproducing the oral structures of the implants by means of brass analogues inserted into the impression prior to casting (**366**). A trial denture can be constructed on this cast to finalise tooth position.
9. After definition of tooth position, a cast super-structure is constructed, and a precision fit to the mouth achieved (**367**).
10. Tooth position, derived from a pre-implant denture and subsequent trial, is reproduced on the metal framework. Completion follows a final try-in stage, and the finished prosthesis is attached, by means of small screws, to each of the implant copings.

The partially edentulous patient

To date there are few published reports of long-term results of the use of implants in the partially edentulous patient. Some are in progress but include few elderly patients.

As previously indicated, posterior placement of implants of adequate length is inhibited by anatomical features. There seems little reason not to consider their use anteriorly, should an older person present with such tooth loss and it prove impossible to achieve an acceptable result with a conventional partial denture or bridgework.

However, there are some problems with fixed appliances linking natural teeth to osseointegrated implants. These arise because the latter lack the physical mobility provided by the normal periodontal membrane. At least one implant system incorporates a flexible component between implant and fixed prosthesis, which is intended to simulate the mobility differential. However, long-term use involves periodic replacement of the flexible component.

It may be that the use of implant techniques is less likely to be of value for the partially dentate elderly patient (except perhaps where one jaw is edentulous). Not only are problems with conventional partial dentures less often experienced, but also the overdenture option may be more appropriate (**368, 369** and Chapter 10).

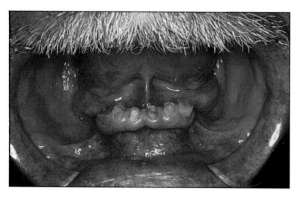

368 Residual natural dentition suitable for overdenture.

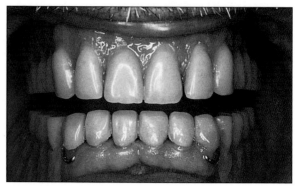

369 Lower overdenture.

References

Branemark, P.-I., Hansson, B.D., Adell, R., Breine, U., Lindstrom, J., Hallen, O. & Ohman, A. 1977. *Osseo-integrated Implants in the Treatment of the Edentulous Jaw – Experience from a Ten-year Period*. Almquist and Wiksell, Stockholm.

Further reading

Naert, I., van Steenburghe, D. & Worthington, P. (eds). 1983. *Osseointegration in Oral Rehabilitation: An Introductory Textbook*. Quintessence, London.

13. Oral Medicine and Pathology

The dentist is having to manage an increasing proportion of patients who have age-related disorders. Individual treatment planning involves not only age changes associated with the teeth but also those occurring within the oral mucosa and salivary glands. In addition to the effects of the physiological ageing process or localised disease it is not unusual for elderly individuals to have symptoms that are due either to systemic illness or long-term medication. This chapter covers the presentation, diagnosis and management of oro-facial conditions which tend to occur in the elderly. The histopathology of some of the conditions will be briefly described and illustrated. The material has been divided into seven categories:

- Normal structures and developmental lesions.
- Infections.
- White patches and oral cancer.
- Dermatoses and pigmented disorders.
- Salivary gland disease.
- Oro-facial pain.
- Oral manifestations of systemic disease.

Normal structures and developmental lesions

Elderly individuals frequently become concerned about the appearance of areas of their oral mucosa and seek the advice of their dental or medical practitioner. Their concern may be initiated by onset of coincidental oral discomfort or the diagnosis of oral cancer in a relative or friend. Mucosal structures which may be thought to represent disease in these circumstances are described below.

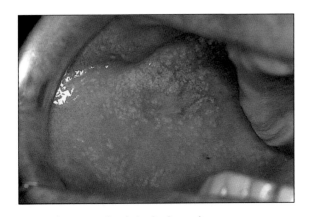

370 Sebaceous glands in the buccal mucosa.

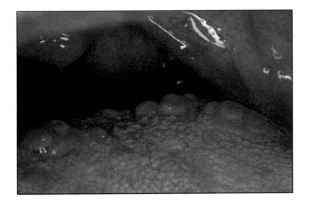

Sebaceous glands

Sebaceous glands (**370**) (Fordyce's spots) are present within the oral mucosa of all individuals to some degree; however, they may become more numerous and obvious with age. The clinical appearance of these glands is sufficiently characteristic for a diagnosis to be made and management should consist of reassurance.

Lingual papillae

The appearance of papillae of the tongue (**371, 372**), in particular the circumvallate (dorsal surface at junction of the anterior two-thirds and one-third) and foliate (lateral surface at junction of anterior two-thirds and posterior one-third) can cause concern. The normal nature of these structures should be explained to the patient. Occasionally, these papillae become inflamed and the use of a topical antiseptic mouthwash such as chlorhexidine can help resolve any symptoms.

371 Circumvallate papillae of the tongue.

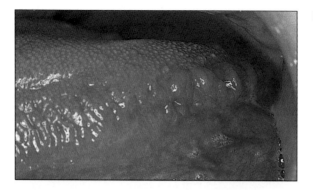

372 Foliate papillae of the lateral surface of the tongue.

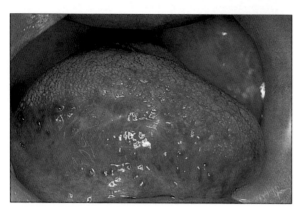

373 Lingual varicosities.

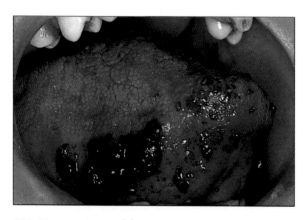

374 Haemangioma of the tongue.

Lingual varicosities

The veins of the ventral surface of the tongue are relatively superficial and can become prominent in later life (**373**). No treatment is required, but patients who become worried about the appearance of these vessels should be reassured.

Haemangioma

True neoplasms of blood vessels are uncommon (**374, 375**), although there has been a relative increase in incidence in recent years as a result of the development of Kaposi's sarcoma (an endothelial neoplasm) in HIV-positive individuals. The majority of haemangioma are congenital malformations of blood vessels which, although present from birth, may become more noticeable in later life. The vascular nature of the lesion can be confirmed clinically by the phenomenon of blanching when held under pressure against a glass slide. A solitary small haemangioma may be excised under local anaesthesia but more extensive and multiple lesions should be referred for specialist treatment, which will usually consist of cryotherapy, embolisation or surgery.

Although frequently described as either cavernous or capillary, many haemangiomas demonstrate both features (**375**). In the top right, thin-walled blood-filled vascular spaces associated with cavernous lesions are present, and in the bottom left, the endothelial cell-rich field typifies a capillary haemangioma.

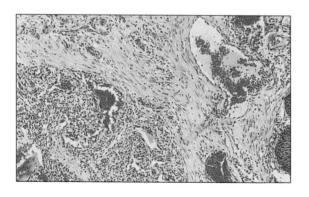

375 Histology of haemangioma; haematoxylin + eosin (H+E) stain.

Geographic tongue (benign migratory glossitis)

Geographic tongue is a condition characterised by irregular erythematous patches surrounded by white margins on the dorsum and lateral margins of the tongue (**376, 377**). Affected areas can resolve within a few days or be persistent. Geographic tongue can be asymptomatic, although most patients complain of discomfort when eating hot or spicy foods. In addition, exacerbation of symptoms has been associated with psychological factors, in particular depression. Diagnosis can usually be made without difficulty from the clinical history and examination, although if doubt exists biopsy should be performed. At the present time the cause of geographic tongue is unknown but it has been associated with zinc deficiency and symptoms may improve following zinc therapy.

The histopathology (**377**) may be indistinguishable from psoriasis, and is characterised by parakeratosis, oedema of the superficial epithelium and lamina propria and an irregular acanthosis that typically includes long square-ended epithelial downgrowths. Chronic candidosis, although usually accompanied by a dense inflammatory infiltrate, may be histologically similar and is excluded by the failure to identify *Candida* hyphae with the periodic acid–Schiff (PAS) reaction.

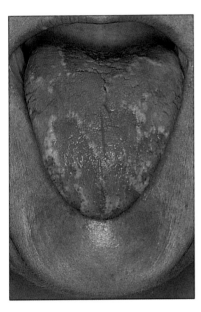

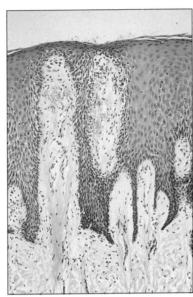

376 Geographic tongue.

377 Histology of geographic tongue (H+E).

Coated tongue

A coating consisting of desquamated epithelial cells and debris often builds up on the dorsal surface of the tongue in debilitated or elderly patients (**378**). If this occurs the surface should be cleaned by instructing the patient to brush their tongue vigorously .

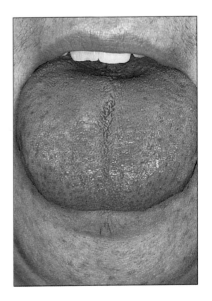

378 Coated tongue.

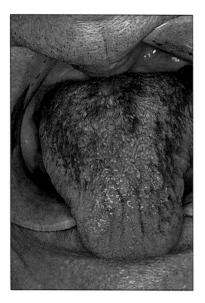

379 Black hairy tongue.

Black hairy tongue

Black hairy tongue (**379**) develops as a result of elongation of the filiform papillae on the dorsal surface of the tongue which subsequently become pigmented. The cause of the condition is unknown but smoking and iron therapy are believed to be contributing factors. Management is as for coated tongue.

Recurrent aphthous stomatitis

Although recurrent aphthous stomatitis (**380**) predominantly affects young adults it can occur at any age. Diagnosis is made by clinical history and appearance of the ulceration.

Initial management should include exclusion of nutritional deficiency, which may be a contributing factor in the elderly. Topical steroids and antiseptic mouthwashes help reduce symptoms, although recurrent aphthous stomatitis can remain troublesome for many years.

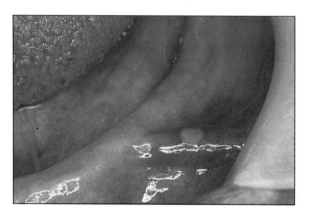

380 Recurrent apthous stomatitis.

Traumatic ulceration

The oral mucosa like any other tissue may suffer from traumatic injury (**381–383**). The most frequent sources of intra-oral trauma are ill-fitting dentures, sharp surfaces on teeth and fractured restorations. Alternatively, the patient may be aware of accidentally biting the buccal mucosa or tongue during eating. The suspected cause of trauma should be eliminated and the ulceration should be seen to resolve within 7–10 days. Ulcers that persist longer than this period of time should undergo biopsy to exclude malignancy. Any area of ulceration that develops in a pre-existing area of smoking-induced keratosis should arouse suspicion of oral malignancy.

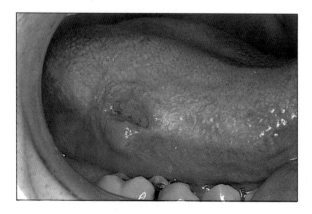

381 Traumatic ulceration caused by a denture.

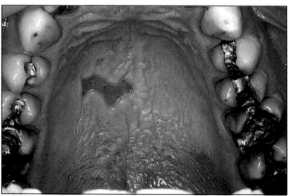

382 Traumatic ulceration of the palate.

The ulcerated mucosa (**383**) is both acute and chronically inflamed, with fibrin clearly identifiable in the surface layers. Adjacent epithelium here shows reactive hyperplasia, but cellular atypia is minimal. Foci of bacterial plaque, which frequently accompany frictional keratosis, are present on the surface.

Denture-induced hyperplasia

The persistent wearing of an ill-fitting denture can induce a hyperplastic reaction within the oral mucosa (**384–386**). This condition is often seen as folds of epithelium in the buccal sulcus, labial sulcus, lingual sulcus or at the junction of the hard and soft palate in relation to the periphery of the denture. Less frequently a leaf-like lesion or multiple raised nodules may appear in the palate. If chronic trauma is suspected then some improvement may be gained by modification of the denture, provision of a tissue conditioner and ensuring that the patient removes the prosthesis at night. Remaining excess tissue should be removed surgically prior to the provision of new dentures.

In long-standing denture-induced hyperplasia (**386**), the proliferation of both epithelium and (mainly) fibrous tissue is an adaptive physiological response, so that apart from some mild irregular acanthosis of the epithelium, the tissues usually appear quite normal. A moderate, patchy, chronic inflammatory response may also be present.

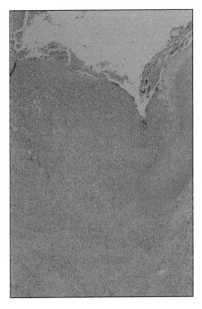

383 Histology of traumatic ulceration (H+E).

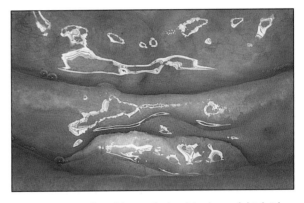

384 Denture induced hyperplasia of the lower labial ridge.

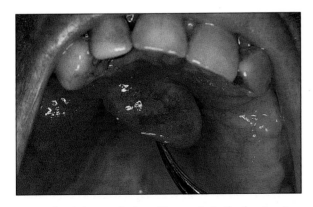

385 Palatal denture induced hyperplasia (leaf pattern).

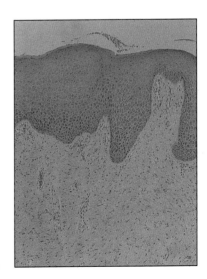

386 Histology of denture induced hyperplasia (H+E).

171

Infections

Elderly patients are prone to the development of opportunistic oral infections, either as a result of diminished efficiency of the host immune defence system or as a secondary effect of an underlying systemic disease.

Tuberculosis

Tuberculosis in the oral cavity is now extremely rare (**387**), although it may still be seen as ulceration of the dorsum of the tongue in patients with open pulmonary disease. However, evidence of previous infection may be seen in elderly patients in the form of calcified lymph nodes which appear as radio-opacities on oro-facial radiographs.

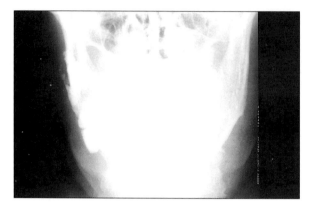

387 Calcified tuberculous lymph nodes.

Candidosis

Approximately 40% of the population harbour *Candida* within their mouth as part of the healthy commensal oral microflora. However, a number of factors (**Table 51**) may predispose to proliferation of these organisms which, in turn, can produce clinical disease. Oral candidosis is traditionally regarded as occurring in four types, all of which are seen in the elderly, although newer forms of candidosis are being described in relation to infection with HIV. Diagnosis of candidosis can be confirmed either by staining of a smear or microbial culture of a swab taken from lesional tissue. Treatment consists of elimination of known local or systemic predisposing factors and the provision of topical antifungal agents. Systemic antifungal agents have recently become available and these may be required in some cases.

Table 51. Factors in the elderly which may predispose to oral candidosis.

Persistent denture wearing
Mucosal irritation
Xerostomia
Malnutrition
Iron deficiency
Vitamin B_{12} deficiency
Maturity onset diabetes mellitus
Hypothyroidism
Leukaemia
Agranulocytosis
High carbohydrate diet
Drug therapy: Antibiotics
Corticosteroids
Immunosuppressives
Cytotoxics

Acute pseudomembraneous candidosis (thrush)

This form of candidosis is characterised by the development of widespread creamy yellow patches within the mouth, which can be wiped off to expose an underlying erythematous mucosa (**388, 389**). It has been reported that pseudomembraneous candidosis occurs in up to 10% of elderly individuals.

388 Acute pseudo-membraneous candidosis of the soft palate.

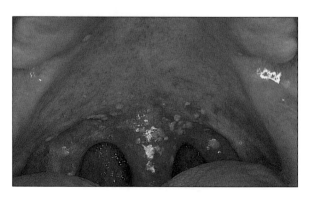

Rapid confirmation of acute pseudomembraneous candidosis may be carried out at the chairside by making a direct smear of the lesion onto a sterile glass slide and either fixing by gentle heating, or by using a commercially available spray-fix. The fixed specimen may then be stained by the PAS reaction and viewed wet within a few minutes of sampling.

Clusters of purple/red candidae spores and pseudohyphae of *Candida albicans* are seen here (in **389**) against pale counter-stained desquamated epithelial cells.

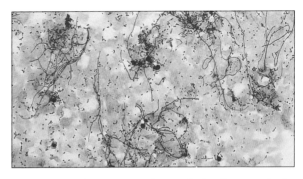

389 Candidal spores and pseudo-hyphae; periodic acid–Schiffs' (PAS) stain.

Acute erythematous (atrophic) candidosis

This is the least common form of oral candidosis which presents as the name implies as the acute development of erythematous areas of the oral mucosa (**390**). Onset of symptoms is often related to the provision of antibiotic or corticosteroid therapy. Unlike the other forms of candidosis the acute erythematous form is painful.

Chronic hyperplastic candidosis

Chronic candidal infection may produce hyperplastic lesions within the oral mucosa (**391**). This can occur at any intraoral site but is characteristically seen bilaterally in the commissure regions of the buccal mucosa. Smoking is a recognised predisposing factor and this form of candidosis is associated with a risk of carcinomatous change. Treatment of chronic hyperplastic candidosis may require the use of systemic antifungal agents.

Histopathological sections characteristically show acanthotic and frequently hyperparakeratotic stratified squamous epithelium, containing abundant PAS-positive *Candida* hyphae (**392**).

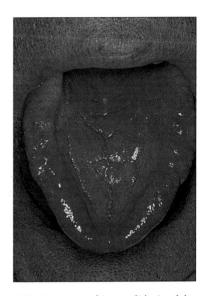

390 Acute atrophic candidosis of the tongue.

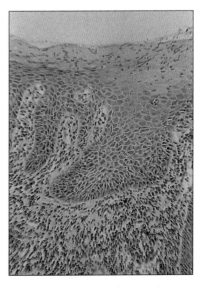

392 Histology of chronic hyperplastic candidosis (PAS).

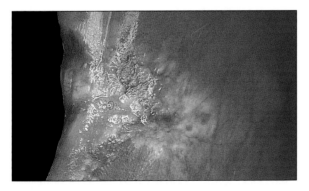

391 Chronic hyperplastic candidosis.

Although most evident in the surface layers, the hyphae may frequently be identified deep in the epithelium. A dense juxta-epithelial mixed chronic inflammatory infiltrate is present, except in immunocompromised patients, when the infiltrate may be minimal.

Chronic erythematous (atrophic) candidosis

This is the most frequently occurring type of oral candidosis (**393**) and it has been suggested that it develops in as many as 50% of individuals with dentures, especially if these are worn both day and night. Clinically, the mucosal changes are limited to the areas of mucosa underlying the denture.

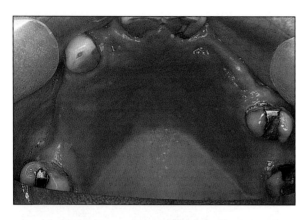

393 Chronic atrophic candidosis.

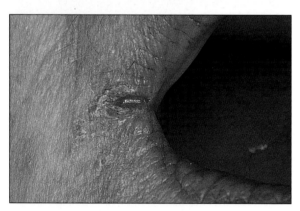

394 Angular cheilitis.

Angular cheilitis

Angular cheilitis is an extremely common clinical condition characterised by the presence of erythema, discomfort and crusting of the angles of the mouth (**394, 395**). The condition represents infection by *Candida* or staphylococci, either alone or in combination. The chronic reservoir of candidal infection in the elderly is often an upper denture that is worn continuously. The anterior nares is likely to be the source of staphylococci. Provision of appropriate topical antimicrobial agents and instruction on adequate denture hygiene, including placement of the prosthesis in dilute hypochlorite solution at night, usually leads to resolution. In prolonged cases the presence of an underlying systemic disease, in particular nutritional deficiency, should be excluded.

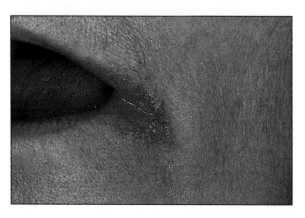

395 Angular cheilitis with extensive crusting.

Shingles (Herpes zoster)

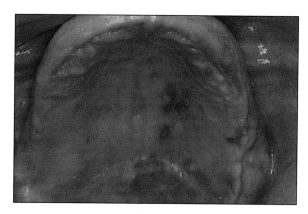

396 Intra-oral *Herpes zoster* infection.

Shingles is a troublesome problem for elderly patients and develops as a result of reactivation of the *Varicella zoster* virus acquired during childhood chickenpox (**396, 397**). Severe unilateral pain affecting one division of the trigeminal nerve is often the first symptom and this is followed within 24–48 h by the appearance of cutaneous and mucosal vesicles. The unilateral and well-delineated distribution of the lesions makes diagnosis straightforward. Treatment should involve systemic acyclovir therapy for at least 10 days, since this approach leads to a rapid resolution of symptoms and is likely to reduce the risk of post-herpetic neuralgia. *Herpes zoster* occurs in greater frequency in patients with malignant disease such as Hodgkin's disease, chronic lymphatic leukaemia, lymphoma and multiple myloma and may occasionally be a presenting sign.

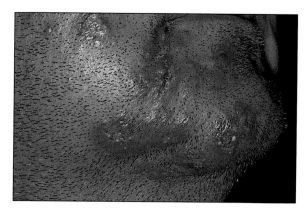

397 *Herpes zoster* infection of the face.

White patches and oral cancer

White patches are frequently found as a coincidental finding during the examination of the oral mucosa of elderly patients. The vast majority of these patches represent benign conditions, but some are associated with the potential for malignant change and the development of oral cancer. Accurate diagnosis and management of any white patch affecting the oral mucosa is therefore essential.

Traumatic keratosis

Chronic low-grade trauma will produce hyperkeratosis of the oral epithelium and this will be seen clinically as a white patch of the mucosa (**398–400**). Eating may produce this appearance in areas of the mouth where missing teeth have not been replaced by fixed or removable prostheses. Elderly patients often find the wearing of a full lower denture difficult and therefore it is not uncommon to find traumatic white patches along the lower edentulous ridge. Irritation caused by smoking may also produce white patches on the oral mucosa, particularly within the palate. Treatment of traumatic keratosis consists of eliminating the suspected aetiological factor and ensuring clinical resolution. Any lesion that persists for longer than 2 weeks or develops ulceration should be biopsied to exclude the presence of carcinoma.

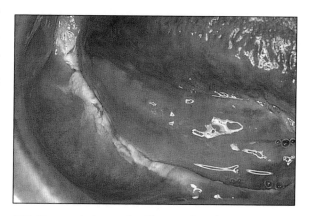

398 Traumatic keratosis of lower edentulous ridge.

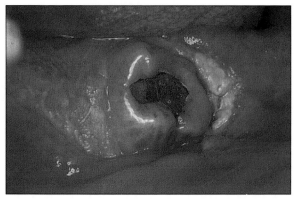

399 Palatal traumatic keratosis.

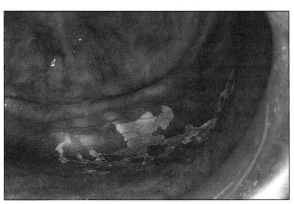

400 Traumatic keratosis.

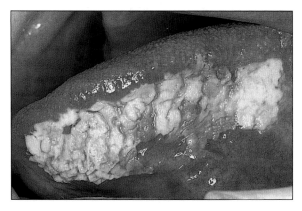

401 Leukoplakia of lateral border of tongue.

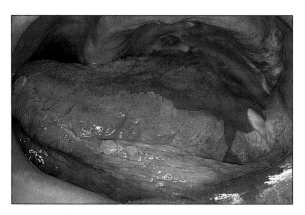

402 Extensive lingual and floor of mouth leukoplakia.

Leukoplakia

Leukoplakia (**401–403**) is a clinical term that is applied to an area of mucosa which presents as 'a white patch that cannot be characterised clinically or pathologically as any other disease'. Leukoplakia is believed to be present in approximately 1–2% of the population in the United Kingdom, although much higher incidences are found in other locations such as the Indian subcontinent. The extent of leukoplakia can vary from a small localised lesion to multiple areas of widespread involvement. The presence of any dysplasia within a white patch cannot be determined clinically and therefore biopsy for histopathological examination must be performed. Subsequent treatment will depend on the degree of any dysplasia. Some consider that severely dysplastic lesions should be treated as carcinoma (see below) while mild or moderate dysplasia may be treated more conservatively. Known predisposing factors such as tobacco, alcohol, nutritional deficiency and oral candidosis should be eliminated and long-term follow-up arranged.

Clinically presenting as leukoplakia of the buccal mucosa, the histology of this white patch shows

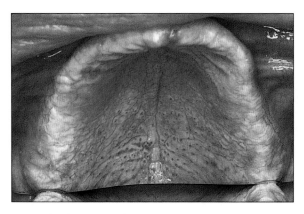

403 Leukoplakia of the lower edentulous ridge.

hyperorthokeratosis and mild dysplasia of the epithelium (**404**). The dysplasia is characterised by frequent hyperchromatic basal cells, and frequent nuclear and cytoplasmic pleomorphism of basal and prickle cells. A moderate chronic inflammatory cell infiltrate is present, mainly confined to the lamina propria. This section (**405**) shows severely dysplastic, grossly hyperparakeratotic atrophic buccal epithelium. There is gross nuclear and cytoplasmic

pleomorphism, loss of desmosomal attachments, foci of early keratinisation, and loss of cell polarity and stratification. Thin, spindle-shaped keratinocytes are present in areas of liquifactive degeneration. Such areas of severe dysplasia may arise *de novo*, or may be found adjacent to a squamous cell carcinoma. Multiple levels for histological examination are therefore desirable.

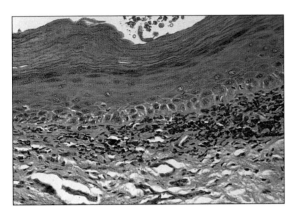

404 Histology of oral mucosa showing mild dysplasia (H+E).

405 Histology of oral mucosa showing severe dysplasia (H+E).

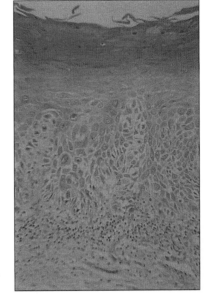

Erythroplakia

Erythroplakia (**406**) is a clinically descriptive term that may be applied to 'a red patch that cannot be characterised clinically or pathologically as any other disease'. Erythroplakia has a greater likelihood of developing into oral carcinoma than

leukoplakia and therefore biopsy is also mandatory. Further management will depend on the severity of dysplasia, as determined histologically.

In this section (**407**) the buccal epithelium shows nuclear hyperchromatism, increased nuclear

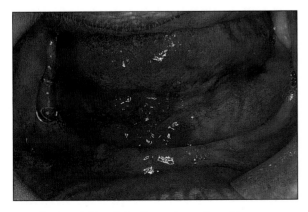

406 Erythroplakia of the floor of mouth and tongue.

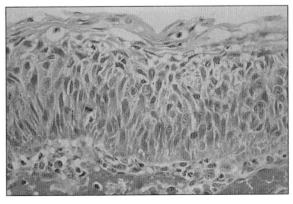

407 Histology of carcinoma *in situ* (H+E).

to cytoplasm ratio and nuclear pleomorphism. Mitoses may be identified within the prickle cell layer, and there is a loss of polarity of the basal cells as well as a diminished intercellular adhesion. These changes extend throughout the depth of the epithelium. Such extreme severity of dysplasia may be termed carcinoma *in situ*.

Squamous cell carcinoma

Squamous cell carcinoma (**408–410**) is a good example of an age-related disease, with 85% of cases in the United Kingdom occurring in individuals over 50 years of age. Although the overall incidence of oral cancer is low compared with other human cancers the mortality rate is quite high, with only 50% of patients surviving longer than 5 years. Many aetiological factors have been proposed for oral cancer but tobacco, alcohol and nutritional deficiency appear to be most important. Once diagnosed histologically, treatment consists of surgery and/or radiotherapy, depending on the extent of the lesion and the general health of the patient. Early diagnosis of small lesions is believed to greatly improve outcome and therefore elderly patients should be examined regularly and any suspicious area of mucosa investigated. Long-term follow-up is required to monitor either recurrence at the primary site or development of further lesions.

The ulcerated keratinising squamous cell carcinoma in **411** arises from buccal epithelium. It is invading upon a broad front and is accompanied by a dense chronic inflammatory infiltrate. The degree of cellular differentiation is only one of several factors (e.g. size, site, metastatic spread, age of the patient), indicative of prognosis and a well-differentiated squamous cell carcinoma, as illustrated here, should not be regarded, purely on histological grounds, as any less serious than an anaplastic tumour.

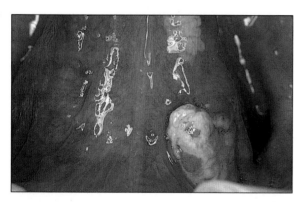

408 Squamous cell carcinoma of the ventral surface of the tongue.

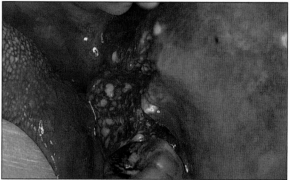

409 Squamous cell carcinoma arising from the retro-molar pad region of the mandible.

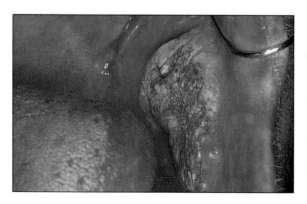

410 Squamous cell carcinoma of the buccal mucosa.

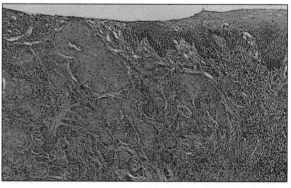

411 Histology of ulcerated keratinising squamous cell carcinoma of the buccal mucosa (H+E).

Skin grafts

Anatomical defects created by surgical removal of extensive soft tissue lesions within the mouth are often repaired using skin grafts (**412**). Clinically, a graft will appear as a white patch with well-defined margins and diagnosis can be confirmed by questioning the patient on previous surgery. It is important to know if the patient received the graft as part of the management of oral cancer since such an individual would be at a high risk of developing further primary oral cancers.

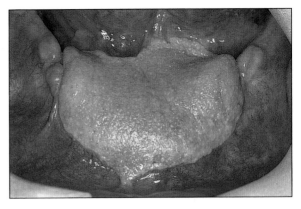

412 Skin graft to lower edentulous ridge.

Dermatoses and pigment disorders

The skin and oral mucosa share a common embryological development and therefore it is not surprising that a number of disease processes affect both sites. Pigmentation of the oral mucosa is often racial, although changes are not uncommon in Caucasians. Factors that may predispose to increased pigmentation include smoking, drug therapy, systemic disease and the presence of malignancy.

Lichen planus

Lichen planus is a chronic inflammatory condition of unknown cause (**413–416**), which is relatively common in patients after middle age. The oral presentation is variable and different subtypes (reticular, erosive, plaque-like and atrophic) have been described. However, distinction between such subtypes is probably not necessary clinically since only symptomatic patients require treatment. Diagnosis is straightforward but mucosal biopsy should be performed if doubt exists. Treatment is based on the use of steroids given either topically, intralesionally or systemically, depending on the severity and extent of involvement.

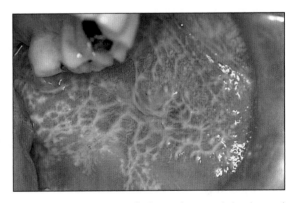

413 Reticular pattern lichen planus of the buccal mucosa.

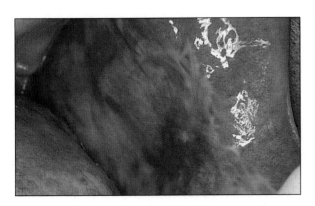

414 Atrophic lichen planus of the buccal mucosa.

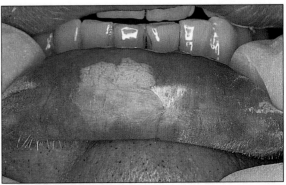

415 Plaque-like lichen planus of the lower labial mucosa and lip.

Major histological features of lichen planus include hyperkeratosis, a distinctive saw-tooth profile to the epithelium, with arching of the papillary corium and a juxta-epithelial dense band of mononuclear cells. The basal layer may be indefinable owing to an intercellular oedema known as liquifactive degeneration (**417**).

416 Erosive lichen planus of the tongue.

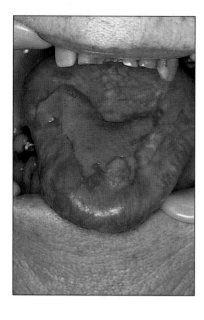

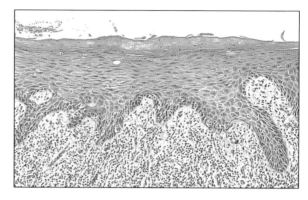

417 Histology of lichen planus of oral mucosa (H+E).

Mucous membrane pemphigoid

Mucous membrane pemphigoid (MMP) mainly affects elderly women and the mouth is often the first site of involvement, with subsequent lesions within the eyes or mucous membranes of the nose, larynx and oesophagus (**418**). Although mucous membrane pemphigoid is a submucosal bullous disorder, intact bullae or vesicles are rarely seen intra-orally since they rupture early to leave areas of erosion or ulceration. Diagnosis can be made by routine histopathological examination, although immunofluorescence techniques are most helpful. Topical and systemic steroids, depending on severity of involvement will usually successfully control disease activity. An ophthalmic opinion should be obtained for all patients found to have mucous membrane pemphigoid, since scarring corneal lesions can develop and the condition is associated with the development of glaucoma.

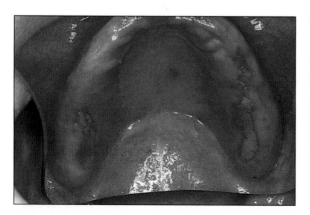

418 Mucous membrane pemphigoid of the palate.

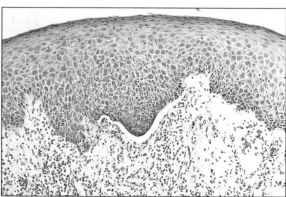

419 Histology of mucous membrane pemphigoid of oral mucosa (H+E).

In mucous membrane pemphigoid, the salient feature is the separation of the full thickness of epithelium from the lamina propria to form a sub-epithelial bulla (**419**). In up to 80% of cases, immunofluorescence can detect C3 deposition in the basement membrane zone (**420**). Circulating antibodies are not usually detected.

Pemphigus

Pemphigus (**421**), a rare but serious vesiculo-bullous disorder, exists in a number of forms, the most common being pemphigus vulgaris which is characterised by lesions on the skin and mucous membranes. The oral cavity may be the site of first involvement and early diagnosis can prevent lesions occurring on the skin. Diagnosis is made by routine histopathological examination of biopsy material, combined with immunofluorescence techniques. Treatment is based on the use of systemic cortico-steroids in combination with the immunomodulatory drug azathioprine. Therapy is life-long and therefore patients may suffer from the consequences of receiving long-term corticosteroid treatment.

Pemphigus vulgaris is characterised histologically by suprabasal splitting of the epithelium, as it is the interepithelial desmosomal cell attachments that are destroyed and not the hemidesmosomal cellular attachment to the basement membrane zone. Loss of intercellular attachment leads to intra-epithelial vesicles containing rounded acantholytic cells floating around in the vesicular fluid (**422**). IgG deposition may be detected along the margins of intact and floating epithelial cells (**423**).

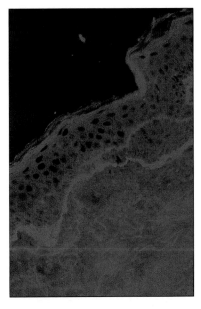

420 Histology of immunofluorescent detection of C3 in the basement membrane zone in mucous membrane pemphigoid.

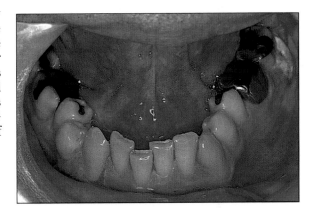

421 Pemphigus.

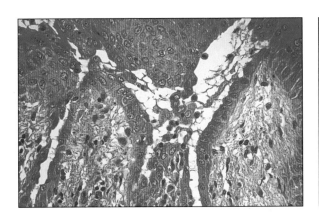

422 Histology of pemphigus vulgaris (H+E).

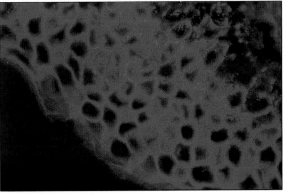

423 Histology of immunofluorescent detection of IgG in pemphigus vulgaris.

181

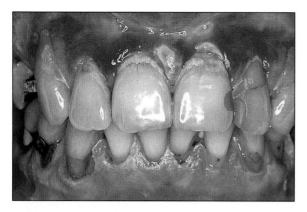

Desquamative gingivitis

Desquamative gingivitis is a clinical term rather than a diagnosis which is used to describe erythematous changes in the gingivae that may arise in forms of lichen planus, mucous membrane pemphigoid and pemphigus (**424**). Desquamative gingivitis responds well to topical steroids.

424 Desquamative gingivitis.

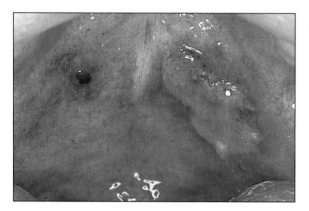

425 Angina bullosa haemorrhagica.

Angina bullosa haemorrhagica

Angina bullosa haemorrhagica is a condition that is characterised by the rapid development of a blood-filled blister at the junction of the hard and soft palate, although it may occur at any oral site (**425**). The bulla ruptures within 12–24 h to leave an area of ulceration that heals spontaneously within 7–10 days. If the presence of thrombocytopenia has been excluded then the patient requires no active treatment other than reassurance.

Smoking-induced pigmentation

Smoking of tobacco stimulates melanocyte activity, which results in diffuse brown pigmentation of oral mucosa, especially in the buccal mucosa and soft palate (**426**). Biopsy may be required to exclude the presence of malignant melanoma. Once diagnosed no treatment is required other than encouraging the patient to stop smoking.

Melanotic pigmentation is an occasional feature of severe hyperkeratosis. It is believed that this is a reaction of the melanocytes to chronic irritation, with possibly an associated dysfunction in the transfer and/or uptake of melanin from melanocytes to keratocytes. This is suggested since much of the melanin is present in sub-epithelial macrophages, having probably leaked out of melanocytes or basal cells (melanin incontinence). At present this pigmentation is considered to have no diagnostic or prognostic significance (**427**).

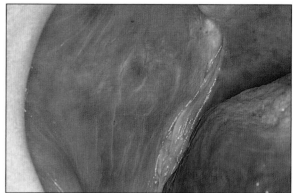

426 Smoking-induced pigmentation of the buccal musosa.

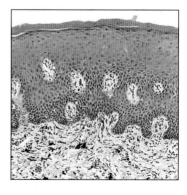

427 Histology of melanotic pigmentation of the oral mucosa.

Melanotic macule

Melanotic macule presents either as single or multiple areas of pigmentation (**428**). Diagnosis should be confirmed by biopsy and thereafter no active treatment is required.

Histologically, these completely benign lesions are characterised by an increase in the amount of melanin in the basal keratinocytes and in the occasional macrophage (melanophage) in the lamina propria (**429**).

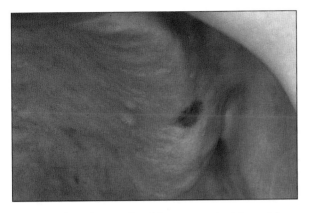

428 A melanotic macule of the upper edentulous ridge.

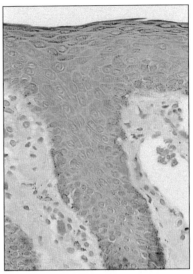

429 Histology of melanotic macule (H+E).

Lentigo

Lentigo is a rare condition with a similar presentation to melanotic macule (**430**). Histological examination of biopsy material is essential since a high percentage of areas of lentiginous change will ultimately develop into malignant melanoma.

This pre-malignant lesion may present as a pigmented macule, most frequently occurring in the palate. Histology shows replacement of basal melanocytes by vacuolated malignant melanocytes, which are frequently spindle-shaped. The epithelium is usually atrophic, with no significant inflammatory infiltrate in the lamina propria (**431**).

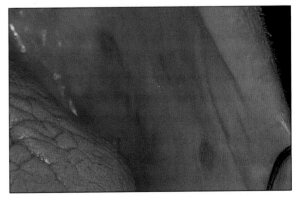

430 Lentigo of the buccal mucosa.

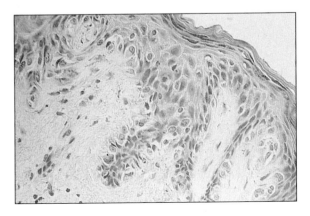

431 Histology of lentigo of the oral mucosa (H+E).

Malignant melanoma

Although a common neoplasm of skin, malignant melanoma is rare in the oral cavity (**432**). If it does occur intra-orally then the maxillary alveolar ridge and palate are the sites most frequently affected. The tumour presents as a discrete deeply pigmented area, often arising within a more extensive region of pigmentation. Diagnosis is achieved by biopsy and treatment consists of radical surgery but the 5-year survival rate is still poor.

Malignant melanomas may not always be heavily pigmented. Histologically, the tumour may present as sheets of epithelioid cells indistinguishable by routine staining from either a poorly differentiated squamous cell carcinoma, or a diffuse large-cell lymphoma. In the section shown in **433** epithelioid cells are well demonstrated, but an occasional pigmented cell supports the clinical prognosis of malignant melanoma. Confirmation may come from either immunocytochemistry (NIKC3 and S100 positive), or electron microscopy demonstrating the presence of melanosomes.

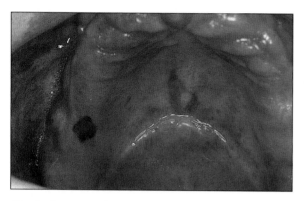

432 Malignant melanoma of the upper edentulous ridge.

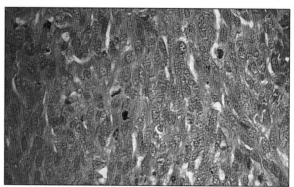

433 Histology of intra-oral malignant melanoma.

Amalgam tattoo

Introduction of amalgam into the oral tissues may occur during dental restorative procedures or at the time of tooth extraction and this may subsequently, sometimes after many months or years, produce discrete areas of mucosal pigmentation (**434**). Clinical diagnosis is supported by evidence on radiographs of radiopaque material, but biopsy should be undertaken. No active treatment is required.

Histologically, the pigment is present as widely dispersed fine brownish or black granules, or as solid fragments of varying size that, when large, may be detected on radiographs. The pigment granules may be scattered haphazardly, but are often associated with collagen and elastic fibres and basement membrane zones (**435**).

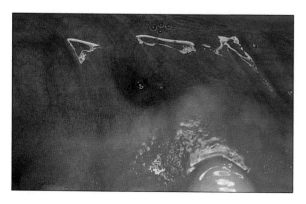

434 Amalgam tattoo of the labial mucosa.

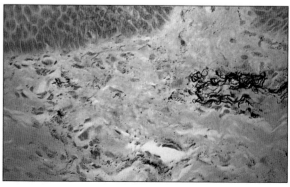

435 Histology of amalgam tattoo (H+E).

Salivary gland disease

Salivary gland disorders may involve major or minor glands, giving rise to localised or generalised effects on salivary tissue.

Xerostomia

A dry mouth is a frequent complaint of the elderly, although clinical examination often fails to reveal any abnormality in the volume of saliva (**436**). The major causes of reduced salivary flow include: Sjögren's syndrome, side effects of drug therapy (**Table 52**) and chronic anxiety or depression.

Lack of saliva causes a number of oral complaints, including difficulty in eating and swallowing, lack of taste, increased incidence of caries and opportunistic candidal infections. Patients with xerostomia should be given artificial saliva substitutes and preventive oral hygiene therapy.

Sjögren's syndrome

Sjögren's syndrome (**437, 438**) is a common condition that is presently divided into two forms, primary and secondary; primary Sjögren's syndrome (previously referred to as sicca syndrome) involves dry mouth and dry eyes, while secondary Sjögren's syndrome consists of dry mouth and/or dry eyes, along with the presence of a connective tissue disorder such as rheumatoid arthritis, systemic lupus erythematosis, systemic sclerosis or primary biliary cirrhosis. Although the presence of reduced salivary and lacrimal flow rates is a good indication of the presence of Sjögren's syndrome the most useful diagnostic test is a labial gland biopsy, although a positive biopsy is not necessarily pathognomonic.

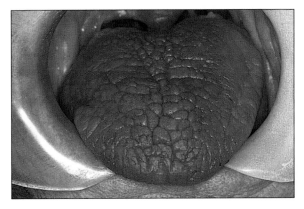

436 Typical appearance of the oral mucosa in elderly person with xerostomia.

Table 52. Types of drugs that may produce xerostomia in the elderly.

Antidepressants
Antihistamines
Anticholinergic drugs
Potent diuretics
Hypotensive agents
Muscle relaxants
Narcotics
Hypnotics
Neuroleptics (major tranquillizers)

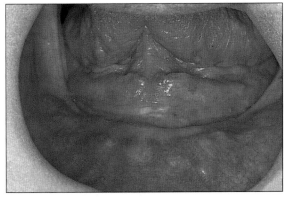

437 Oral mucosa in Sjögren's syndrome.

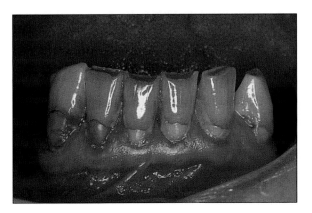

438 High caries incidence in Sjögren's syndrome.

185

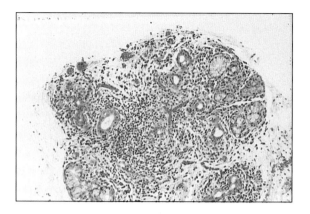

The salient histological features are acinar atrophy, duct dilatation, replacement fibrosis and foci, frequently dense, of periductal or perivascular lymphocytes (**439**). However, Sjögren's syndrome is a clinical diagnosis and these changes are only consistent with the syndrome in the absence of any oral lesions such as major aphthae, the changes beneath which may be identical.

439 Histology of labial glands in Sjögren's syndrome (H+E).

Sialorrhoea

The complaint of excess salivation (**440**) is much less frequent than that of a dry mouth but it may occur in patients with diabetic autonomic neuropathy, Parkinson's disease and cerebral palsy. It is also recognised that patients complaining of excess salivation often have an underlying psychiatric problem.

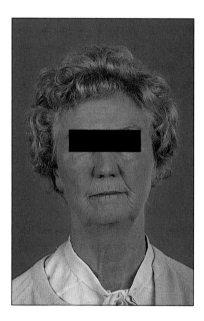

440 This patient has excessive salivation caused by Parkinson's disease.

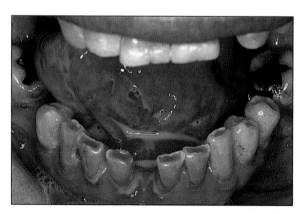

441 Bacterial sialadenitis of the submandibular gland. A purulent discharge is noted from the duct.

Bacterial sialadenitis

The presenting symptoms of bacterial sialadenitis consist of an enlarged painful gland with purulent discharge at the duct orifice (**441**). Microbiological studies have implicated streptococci and strict anaerobes as the organisms most likely to be involved and therefore patients should be prescribed with a broad-spectrum antibiotic such as amoxycillin. Following the resolution of acute infection, the gland should be investigated by sialography for any predisposing factors such as sialoliths, duct strictures or Sjögren's syndrome.

Sialolith and mucous plugs

Sialoliths (calculi, stones) or mucous plugs can form within the duct of the major salivary glands and lead to obstruction of salivary flow (**442**). Obstruction will produce symptoms of gland swelling, especially during eating. Clinical examination and sialography should reveal the nature of the underlying problem. Salivary stones may be removed surgically if situated in the anterior part of the duct, while mucous plugs may be disrupted using lacrimal dilators. Removal of the salivary gland may be necessary if large calculi are present within the gland itself or when there is evidence of gross gland damage.

Intraglandular sialoliths (**443**) may be homogenous or frequently, as illustrated here, have a lamented appearance consistent with slow incremental growth. The ducts within which they occur are dilated, and associated lobules of salivary gland tissue may show varying degrees of atrophy and non-specific sialadenitis.

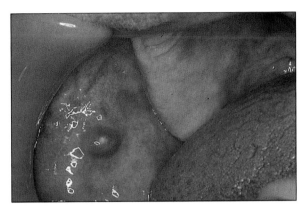

442 Sialolith of the parotid gland duct.

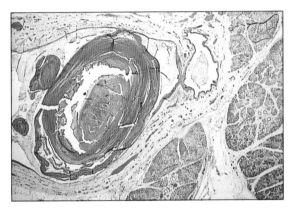

443 Histology of intraglandular sialolith (H+E).

Mucocele

A cyst that develops within a minor salivary gland is termed a mucocele (**444**) and this can arise at any intra-oral site but is seen particularly within the lower lip. Diagnosis is usually obvious from the clinical appearance and history but a haemangioma can occasionally have a similar appearance. Treatment of a mucocele consists of surgical incision.

An incompletely healed traumatised salivary gland duct may permit extravasation of mucus into adjacent soft tissue until tissue pressure terminates the outflow. The cavity formed is not lined by epithelium (**445**).

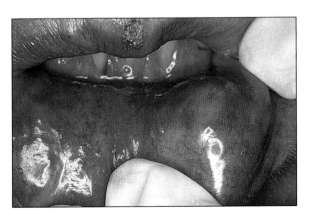

444 Mucocele of lower lip.

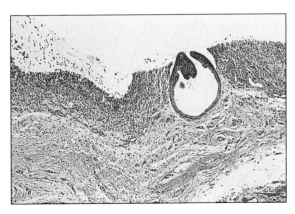

445 Histology of mucocele (H+E).

A higher power view (**446**) of the duct illustrates an inadequate attempt at repair, resulting in mucous extravasation.

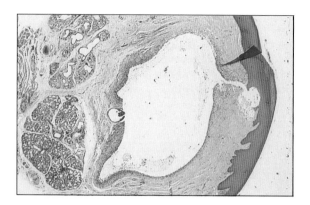

446 High power view of histology of mucocele (H+E).

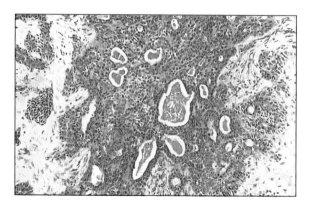

447 Pleomorphic adenoma of the parotid salivary gland.

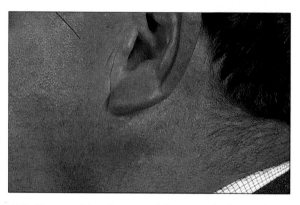

448 Histology of pleomorphic salivary gland (H+E).

Pleomorphic salivary adenoma

Pleomorphic salivary adenoma (PSA) is a benign neoplasm that accounts for the majority of tumours that arise in salivary tissue (**447**). Pleomorphic salivary adenoma is characterised by a slowly enlarging painless swelling of the affected gland, most frequently the parotid. A proportion of cases undergo malignant transformation and may represent carcinoma-ex-PSA. Diagnosis is achieved by biopsy and treatment consists of surgical excision.

The complex intermingling of epithelial components and mesenchymal areas provides a great variety of histological appearances – hence the adjective pleomorphic. Well circumscribed, if not always encapsulated, the tumour contains epithelial components arranged in sheets, clumps and duct-like structures. Both epithelial-duct cells and myoepithelial type cells are present. The intercellular material varies in quantity, being generally less abundant in tumours of the minor rather than the major salivary glands. Qualitatively, it also varies from fibrous delicate tissue to dense, scar-like deposits, frequently containing elastic tissue, but most characteristically as myxoid/chondroid tissue. All these variants of intercellular material may be present in a single tumour (**448**).

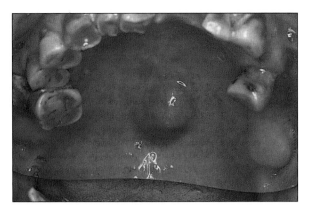

449 Adenoid cystic carcinoma of the palatal minor salivary glands.

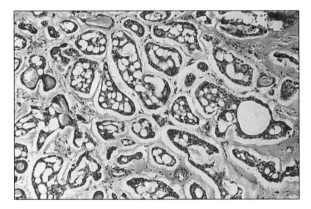

450 Histology of adenoid cystic carcinoma.

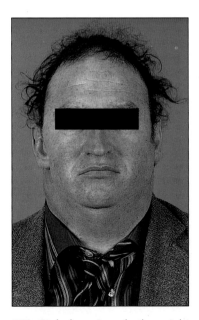

451 Sialadenosis of the right parotid salivary gland.

Adenoid cystic carcinoma

Malignant neoplasms of salivary tissue are relatively more common in minor glands and are characterised by the presence of a slowly enlarging mass, with localised destruction of the surrounding tissues (**449**). Biopsy is diagnostic and treatment involves a wide surgical excision because of the aggressive nature of the condition.

The characteristic feature of this malignant epithelial tumour is the presence of numerous microscopic cyst-like spaces within the epithelial islands, producing a cribriform or 'Swiss cheese' pattern. The spaces are formed by the partial enclosure of areas of stroma or of mucoid materials produced by the tumour epithelium itself, which are deposited adjacent to the stroma. The cells of the epithelial component are predominantly small, uniform polygonal cells with basophilic cytoplasms (**450**).

Sialadenosis

Sialadenosis is a term used to describe a non-inflammatory non-neoplastic persistent swelling of the major salivary glands (**451**). The cause is unknown but alcohol abuse, altered liver function, anorexia, drug therapy and maturity onset diabetes mellitus are all known as predisposing factors which need to be excluded. The presence of sialadenosis may be confirmed histologically, although once diagnosed no localised treatment is required and the degree of swelling may reduce following correction of any underlying systemic disease.

The characteristic histology shows enlargement of the serous acinar cells and slight compression of the duct system by the swollen acini. The nuclei are displaced towards the periphery of the cells. There are no histological features to suggest malignancy and there is an absence of inflammatory reaction (**452**).

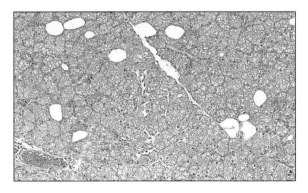

452 Histology of sialadenosis (H+E)

Oro-facial pain

Oro-facial pain is one of the main reasons patients seek dental treatment. In the elderly, the diagnosis of oro-facial pain of non-dental origin can present a considerable clinical problem. A detailed history of symptoms and the nature of the pain is essential to ensure accurate diagnosis and successful treatment.

Burning mouth syndrome

Burning mouth syndrome is a common condition in the elderly, particularly women (**453**). Terms previously used to describe a burning sensation affecting the oral mucosa include stomatopyrosis, glossopyrosis and glossodynia. However, the use of the term burning mouth syndrome is useful since patients can relate to it easily and are reassured by a diagnosis. Burning mouth syndrome is a multifactorial problem involving denture design, deficiency of haematinics, undiagnosed maturity onset diabetes mellitus, parafunctional habits and psychological components such as cancerphobia, anxiety and depression. Clinical examination will fail to reveal any mucosal abnormality and therefore a team approach is required to eliminate all potential aetiological factors.

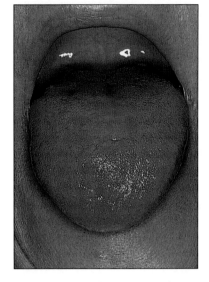

453 Tongue in burning mouth syndrome.

Temporomandibular joint pain

Simplistically, the pattern of temporomandibular joint pain may be divided into joint disease (which is rare) and joint dysfunction (which is extremely common) (**454, 455**). In temporomandibular joint disease there is a structural disorder of the joint and this is likely to be detectable on radiographs. Anatomical abnormalities can be corrected surgically and this often resolves any symptoms. In temporomandibular joint dysfunction, radiographs will fail to demonstrate any abnormality, although clinical examination will usually reveal tenderness of associated musculature and audible clicking on jaw movements. If the patient is dentate then occlusal splint therapy is the most effective treatment. However, many elderly patients are edentulous and therefore an approach using a splint is not possible. Such patients should be provided with adequate partial or full dentures as necessary, although, in the short term, relief of symptoms may be achieved by the provision of a low dose of dothiepin before sleep.

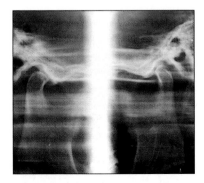

454 Radiograph of temporomandibular joints in patient with temporomandibular joint pain dysfunction.

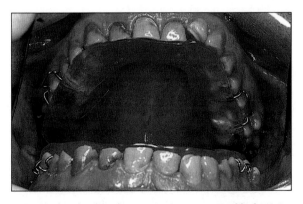

455 Occlusal splint therapy in temporomandibular joint pain dysfunction.

Atypical facial pain

Atypical facial pain is characterised by the presence of an unremitting pain, usually in the maxilla, for which there is no obvious clinical or radiographical cause (**456**). Patients are mostly women who also complain of headache, backache, irritable bowel and itchy skin. Anxiety and depression are likely to be major underlying factors and therefore patients often respond well to dothiepin.

Trigeminal neuralgia

Trigeminal neuralgia is a common cause of facial pain in the elderly (**457**). The nature and history of the symptoms are diagnostic and consist of a recurrent severe lancinating pain that lasts for a few seconds and is limited to one division of the trigeminal nerve. Factors that predispose to the onset of pain include eating, talking and touching the skin of the face. Carbamazepine is the drug of choice and, if correctly used, will successfully alleviate symptoms in the majority of cases. Therapy should be continued for at least 1 year, during which time full blood count and liver function should be monitored at monthly intervals. Surgical intervention should only be considered as a last resort for those patients who do not respond to drug therapy.

Post-herpetic neuralgia

Severe pain is a well-recognised problem following recovery from shingles (**458**). Evidence of previous herpes zoster may be seen as pigmentation of the skin in the affected area. Unfortunately, the pain of post-herpetic neuralgia rarely responds to drug therapy and therefore can present a difficult management problem.

Facial nerve palsy

Acute onset of facial nerve weakness is most often a lower motor neurone lesion referred to as Bell's palsy (**459**). The patient may notice some altered sensation over one side of the face but the main complaint is weakness of the muscle of facial expression owing to VII nerve dysfunction. Clinical signs include a unilateral inability to smile, whistle, close the eye and wrinkle the forehead. Treatment should consist of provision of high-dose systemic steroids and protection of the exposed part of the eye until resolution occurs, which is usually within 7 to 10 days.

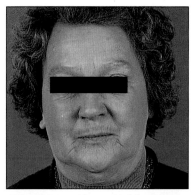

456 Patient with atypical facial pain.

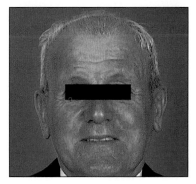

457 Patient with left-sided trigeminal neuralgia.

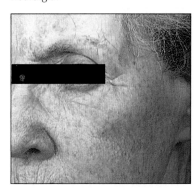

458 Pigmentation in post-herpetic neuralgia patient.

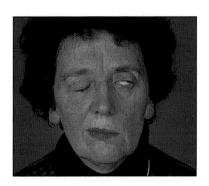

459 Facial nerve palsy.

Oral manifestations of systemic disease

Although the majority of conditions and abnormalities occurring in the mouth are caused by local disease, occasions do arise when signs and symptoms are manifestations of systemic disease or systemic drug therapy. It is not possible in a text of this size to describe the full range of oro-facial manifestations of systemic illnesses and therefore only a selection of those conditions that are seen most frequently in the elderly is presented.

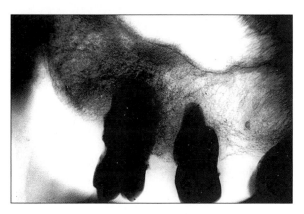

460 Root hypercementosis in Paget's disease.

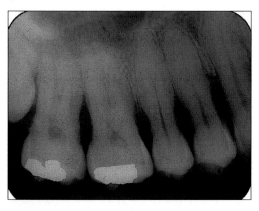

461 This radiograph shows the expansion of tooth roots in Paget's disease.

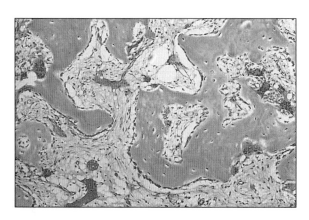

462 Histology of Paget's disease (H+E).

Paget's disease

This condition is of unknown origin, but is probably present in many elderly individuals although only a minority have significant clinical signs and symptoms (**460**). The bones most frequently involved are the sacrum, spine, femur, pelvis and skull. In the jaws, the maxilla is involved more often than the mandible and this may be seen as broadening of the palate and thickening of the alveolar processes. Extraction of teeth in a patient with Paget's disease may be complicated owing to hypercementosis of the roots. Diagnosis is made by blood investigations (raised alkaline phosphatase of bony origin), radiographs (a cotton-wool appearance) or biopsy (mosaic appearance). At present, treatment, if necessary, consists of the provision of calcitonin and diphosphonates.

A feature of Paget's disease of bone affecting the jaws may be hypercementosis, sometimes presenting on a radiograph as a fuzzy expansion of the affected tooth root (**461**). Decalcified histological sections of untreated Paget's provide evidence of rapid bone turnover and osteoblast-rich osteoid and coarse-woven bone being simultaneously resorbed by frequently massive osteoclasts. The interosseous fibrous tissue is usually highly vascular, although the vascularity may diminish as the disease becomes long-standing (**462**). Ground sections of bone from long-standing cases of Paget's may show a mosaic pattern caused by the delineation of reversal lines formed as the bone has been progressively resorbed and laid down.

Diabetes mellitus

Undiagnosed or poorly controlled maturity onset diabetes mellitus may produce a number of oral symptoms including burning mouth syndrome, prolonged candidal infection and altered taste

(463). If an elevated fasting plasma blood glucose is detected then patients should be referred to an appropriate physician. Once adequate glycaemic control has been achieved the oral symptoms usually resolve.

Lupus erythematosis

Lupus erythematosis, an autoimmune disease of unknown cause, can present with a variety of clinical symptoms, depending on the tissues of organs affected (464). Oral lesions of systemic lupus erythematosis and discoid lupus erythematosis are identical and consist of erosive white patches similar to those of lichen planus. Treatment is based on the use of anti-inflammatory agents immunosuppressive therapy and corticosteroids.

The histological features are very variable and diagnosis should not be made on histological criteria alone. The major features that may be present are hyperkeratosis, alternating atrophy and acanthosis, which is sometimes accompanied by keratin-plugging liquifaction of the basal cell layer and a dense infiltrate of chronic inflammatory cells in the lamina propria. The appearances can be similar to those of lichen planus. A useful discriminatory feature may be the presence of deeper perivascular foci of lymphocytes not usually seen in lichen planus (465).

Leukaemia

The acute forms of leukaemia (466) tend to affect young individuals, whereas the chronic types (chronic lymphocytic leukaemia and chronic myeloid leukaemia) are more common in the elderly. Oro-facial changes occurring in chronic leukaemia include gingival swelling, submucosal

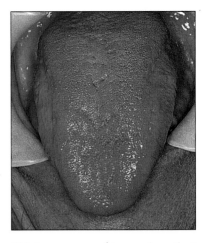

463 Appearance of tongue in patient with poorly controlled maturity onset diabetes.

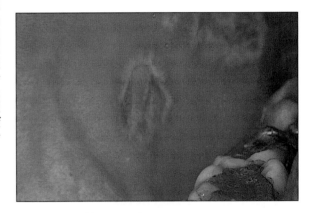

464 Intra-oral lupus erythematosis.

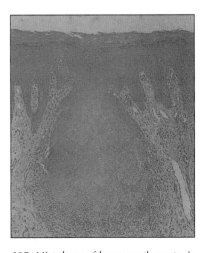

465 Histology of lupus erythematosis (H+E).

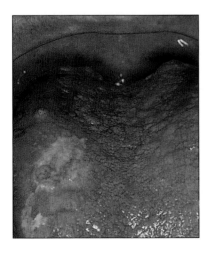

466 Oral ulceration in chronic lymphocytic leukaemia.

petechiae, oral ulceration, atypical viral infections and oral candidosis. Drugs used to treat leukaemia may themselves produce mucosal changes similar to lichenoid reactions. Management of oral lesions consists of maintaining adequate oral hygiene and provision of anti-microbial agents to suppress opportunistic infections.

Lymphoma

Lymphoma consists of a group of neoplasms with varying degrees of malignancy, which may be broadly grouped into Hodgkin's and non-Hodgkin's types (**467, 468**). The elderly are prone to non-Hodgkin's lymphomas which can develop within lymphoid tissue of the salivary glands, especially in patients with Sjögren's syndrome. Treatment is based on the use of radiotherapy and chemotherapy.

With a frequency of about 5% of cases of Sjögren's syndrome, examination of multiple levels of tissue taken from Sjögren's-affected glands is mandatory. The salient feature is an expansion of the lymphoid component to not only totally efface the acini, but to swarm through and obliterate the fibrous interlobular septae. Exclusion of a diffuse non-Hodgkin's lymphoma is then obligatory, and sections must be prepared for immunocytochemical evidence of monoclonicity (**469**).

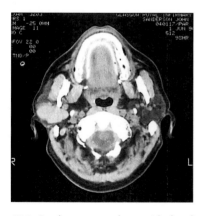

467 Lymphoma of parotid gland

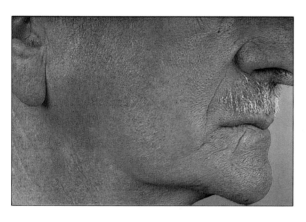

468 Replacement of parotid gland (right) by lymphoma is noted on this C.A.T. scan.

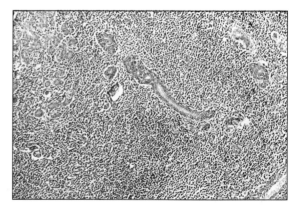

469 Histology of lymphoma in Sjögren's syndrome (H+E).

Lichenoid reaction

A number of drugs given systemically for disease management may produce oral changes that are both clinically and histologically similar to those of lichen planus (**470**). Such lesions are often referred to as lichenoid reactions and are most commonly associated with antihypertensive drugs, non-steroidal anti-inflammatory agents and oral hypoglycaemics. Diagnosis can usually be made by clinical appearance and a history of onset following the prescription of systemic medication. If patients develop significant symptoms then consideration should be given to a change in their drug therapy.

The histological features are essentially those of lichen planus. The section shown in **471** is grossly hyperkeratotic, but atrophic buccal epithelium is accompanied by dense juxta-epithelial band of lymphocytes. Occasionally, the presence of eosinophils, not usually a feature of lichen planus, may suggest a lichenoid reaction, as may the occasional large hyperchromatic basal cell. However, these features are frequently absent and the diagnosis can only be made in conjunction with the clinical findings.

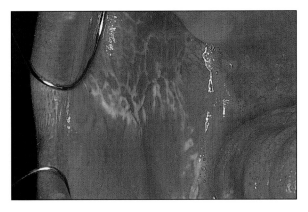

470 Lichenoid reaction of buccal mucosa.

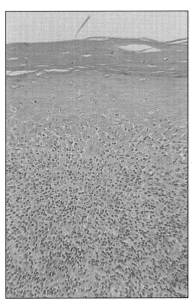

471 Histology of lichenoid reaction (H+E).

Further reading

Eveson, J. & Cawson, R.A. 1987. *A Colour Atlas of Oral Pathology*. William Heinemann, London.

Jones, J.H. & Mason, D.K. (eds). 1990. *Oral Manifestations of Systemic Disease*. Baillière Tindall, London.

Lamey, P.J. & Lewis, M.A.O. 1991. *Oral Medicine in Practice*. British Dental Association, London.

Lewis, M.A.O. & Lamey, P.J. 1994. *Clinical Oral Medicine*. Butterworth, London.

MacFarlane, T.W. & Samaranayake, L.P. 1989. *Clinical Oral Microbiology*. Wright, London.

Millard, H.D. & Mason, D.K. (eds). 1989. *Perspectives on 1988 Workshop on Oral Medicine*. Year Book Medical Publishers, London.

Scully, C. & Cawson, R.A. 1987. *Medical Problems in Dentistry*, 2nd edn. Wright, Bristol.

14. Oral Surgery Considerations

Previous chapters have highlighted demographic changes that present the oral surgeon with an increasing exposure to work with the elderly and to the management problems that they present. Within this demographic group there is great variety; at one extreme the spritely pensioner equally capable of a brisk 5-mile walk as of stoically tolerating a surgical procedure under local anaesthesia; at the other the frail, lonely old lady confused and threatened by the clinical situation. The challenge to the oral surgeon lies first and foremost in assessing the patient as an individual and then considering his or her medical status. The oral surgery is usually the least of the management problems.

Patient assessment

Time spent talking to the elderly is always appreciated and can be used to begin to win the patient's confidence. Clinical, nursing and other ancillary staff all have an important role to play in this small but valuable part of patient management. It is also an opportunity to assess the patient's degree of independence and the availability of help from family, neighbours and social services. This information will be needed later when decisions have to be made regarding treatment plans.

Medical History

A thorough medical history is always important, but even more so in the elderly. They are more likely than the general population to suffer from single or multiple pathologies or to be taking prescribed or over-the-counter medication. Medical problems in the elderly have already been outlined in Chapter 3.

The oral problem and examination

Finally, the oral problem can be considered. This should include detailed enquiries into the nature of the complaint, the degree of pain and disability being suffered and the effect that this has on the patient's day-to-day life.

A thorough inspection of skin, cervical lymph nodes and temporomandibular joints forms the basis of the first part of the examination. The clinician can then turn to the oral cavity and the mucous membranes of the mouth; oro-pharynx should be looked at carefully, followed by a review of the natural dentition and any prosthesis present. Special investigations, in particular the ortho-pantomograph, help to supplement the examination. Hopefully, at this stage a clearer picture of the patient, their medical history and oral problem emerges. Decisions can now be made regarding treatment.

Treatment planning

This is the central issue and is perhaps the most difficult topic to deal with clearly. A decision to perform any operation involves balancing the potential gains from the procedure against the operative risks and possible post-operative complications. If a patient presents with a strangulated hernia or fractured neck of femur the indications for operation are clear and usually outweigh the contra-indications. Oral surgery problems in the elderly are seldom so threatening but it is fair to say that quality of life can be affected. The patient with the fractured mandible or acutely infected retained tooth needs treatment. Equally, procedures to allow comfortable denture wear are of great benefit to the elderly. Consequently, the clinician is drawn into balancing the benefits of treatment against the problems associated with surgery; into this decision comes the inevitable choice between local and general anaesthesia.

General anaesthesia

General anaesthesia presents greater risk to the elderly population than the younger age groups. Operative and postoperative complications usually involve the cardiovascular system with the possibility of deep vein thrombosis, myocardial infarction and heart failure being particular concerns. In addition, postoperative respiratory and urinary tract infections may prove troublesome. Attempts have been made to anticipate risk factors, e.g. Goldman's cardiac risk index in which nine clinical and laboratory findings are scored. The cumulative total then gives an indication of the degree of risk for the patient and this can then be balanced against the indications for surgery.

Analyses such as these are usually applied to patients undergoing major surgery, but the principle holds true for proposed oral procedure. Certainly, if a general anaesthetic is being considered for oral surgery it is sensible to arrange preliminary investigations at the out-patient visit and these include the following:
• Full blood count and haemoglobin examination.

This may show an unexpected anaemia.
• Chest radiograph. In patients over 70 years of age 60% of chest radiographs will show an abnormality and 2.5% will show a neoplastic lesion.
• An electrocardiogram. In the elderly 50%–80% of electrocardiograms will show an abnormality.

It is accepted that these investigations do not necessarily predict postoperative cardiorespiratory problems, but they may reveal previously unsuspected disease and they do form valuable base-line observations should complications arise in the postoperative period. It is essential that a senior anaesthetist has the opportunity to examine the patient preoperatively and review the results of these investigations. Decisions regarding the procedure may then be fully discussed.

General anaesthesia has advantages for the surgeon. It allows more complex procedures to be performed with improved access to the surgical site and the patient benefits by avoiding what might have been a stressful procedure carried out under local anaesthesia.

Local anaesthetic

The use of local anaesthetic avoids, to a large extent, the medical complications associated with general anaesthesia. In suitable patients it is the anaesthetic of choice for simple procedures. The most commonly used agent is lignocaine 2% with 1 in 80 000 adrenalin. It was suggested in the past that adrenalin containing local anaesthetic solutions were contraindicated in patients with known cardiovascular disease. However, recent studies have shown that there are no significant haemodynamic changes with the use of adrenalin and it would therefore seem appropriate to continue using this agent for elderly patients. However, there is the problem of reduced plasma potassium concentrations with the use of adrenalin. This effect is exacerbated in those patients taking non-potassium-sparing diuretics and there is a risk of harmful arrhythmias being produced. It may be that in these patients an alternative local anaesthetic should be used, e.g. Prilocaine with Octapressin.

Local anaesthesia has the advantage of minimising the disturbance to the patient's daily routine and in particular avoids a stay in hospital. As a compromise, it may be possible to arrange a short period of postoperative observation to allow the surgeon to be sure that no medical or surgical complication is likely to develop. These procedures may be stressful for the patient and clear explanation at the preoperative visit, combined with a reassuring manner, go a long way towards minimising patient apprehension.

Common concurrent medical problems

Anticoagulant medication

The elderly may be taking oral anticoagulant drugs which are often prescribed for deep vein thrombosis, poorly controlled atrial fibrillation and patients with prosthetic heart valves. The significance of this medication is twofold. First, its use points to underlying disease that will require further enquiry. Second, the anticoagulant regime will have to be modified before any surgical procedure is undertaken. This should always be discussed with the patient's physician who is responsible for adjusting the anticoagulant dose. An International Normalised Ratio (INR) level of between 2 and 2.5 is appropriate for oral surgery. The patient can resume their normal medication within 24 h of the operation.

Prophylaxis against infective endocarditis

Patients with a history of rheumatic or valvular heart disease, previous infective endocarditis or prosthetic heart valves should receive antibiotic prophylaxis to prevent infective endocarditis following oral surgery procedures. Most prophylactic regimes are based on amoxycillin. The presence of prosthetic heart valves, or a previous episode of infective endocarditis are thought to increase the risk and genta- mycin is then added to the preoperative antibiotic cover. In those patients who are allergic to penicillin or have received it more than once during the month prior to surgery, erythromycin or clinda- mycin are alternatives. It is important to remember that these regimes are frequently updated and a current British National Formulary, or an equivalent, should be consulted if in doubt.

Corticosteroid medication

Some patients may be taking steroid preparations as part of treatment for conditions such as rheumatoid disease. Prednisolone, dexamethasone or beta- methasone are common oral agents and they have the effect of suppressing the normal activity of the adrenal cortex. Consequently, during times of stress, the gland is unable to respond to increased gluco- corticoid demand. Surgery, including oral surgery produces such a demand. Simple procedures under a local anaesthesia can be covered by increasing the usual oral dose on the day of surgery and gradually returning the patient to their normal regime within 48 hours. More major procedures as in-patients will require correspondingly higher doses possibly with the addition of intramuscular or intravenous hydrocortisone.

The diabetic patient

Most elderly diabetic patients will be non-insulin dependent and are controlled by a combination of diet and oral hypoglycaemic agents. This should not present a problem for work under local anaesthetic and the patient should be encouraged to continue with their normal meals and medication. For procedures under general anaesthesia, the oral hypoglycaemic agent can be omitted for the day of surgery.

A few older diabetics will be insulin dependent. Work under general anaesthesia clearly requires a period of starvation and, consequently, carefully controlled fluid and insulin management is required. Once again, work under local anaesthesia does not require any change in the normal diet and insulin regime.

Surgical procedures in the elderly

The maxilla and mandible, as with other bones, lose calcified tissue with age and this has been discussed in Chapter 4. The effect of these changes is generally unhelpful in terms of oral surgery procedures, although not all the odds are stacked against the oral surgeon. Periodontal disease may have advanced sufficiently in some patients to allow the relatively straightforward extraction of many teeth. However, this is not always the case and careful technique, allied to anticipation of problems is most important. This anticipation of difficulties is greatly helped by radiographs and orthopantomograph views of the mandible and maxilla are particularly useful. Not only is the particular surgical question that is being dealt with clarified, but other problems may also become apparent. These may take the form of retained roots and teeth and, although there is seldom any indication for their treatment if asymptomatic, it is part of a thorough examination to be aware of their presence.

Specific oral surgical problems

Removal of teeth and roots

As suggested above, the anticipation of difficulties is important. The radiograph will show root morphology and the extent of any caries. A history of difficult extractions, particularly if combined with radiographic evidence of retained roots, should also act as a warning. A carefully controlled extraction technique is advisable and usually the procedure can be completed within a few minutes. If the extraction is clearly going to be difficult it may be better to consider a surgical approach to the tooth rather than persisting with dental forceps. Retained roots in the jaws are common and only need removal if symptomatic (**472**). Radiographs are required to show the degree of surgical difficulty and if clinically visible, straightforward elevation may be sufficient. Failing this, a simple flap procedure, with or without bone removal, is usually all that is required.

Teeth in the maxillary tuberosity, especially if isolated, present a particular problem. The relative ease of bone fracture and the proximity of the maxillary antrum increase the risk of a fractured tuberosity and oro-antral communication. Radiographs will help indicate difficult root morphology, and the relationship to the maxillary antrum should be clear. Unless the teeth are obviously mobile it is often better to commence their removal as a surgical procedure. This involves the raising of a simple buccal flap and the removal of sufficient buccal bone to allow the relatively atraumatic delivery of the tooth.

This problem is illustrated in **473**. A 70-year-old lady required the removal of her remaining upper teeth prior to the fitting of an immediate upper denture. While attempting the extraction of the

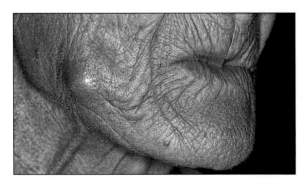

472 Retained lower molar root producing a small buccal abscess.

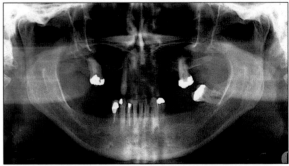

473 Orthopantomograph showing isolated maxillary molar teeth and their close relationship to the maxillary sinus.

upper left second molar the dental practitioner noticed the tuberosity moving and sensibly stopped the procedure. This tooth and the upper right second molar were subsequently removed surgically without further incident and the immediate denture fitted.

Retained wisdom teeth

The retained wisdom tooth presenting late in life is a common problem and **474** shows the typical clinical picture. It may present with acute or chronic infection and often creates difficulties for the denture wearer. The immediate problem can often be solved by simple easing of the prosthesis, but usually removal of the tooth will be required for a long-term solution. Radiographs will give an indication of the root morphology and the expected degree of difficulty of the procedure (**475**). In addition, the relative relationship of the tooth to the inferior dental canal can be seen. If there is any likelihood of damage to the inferior dental nerve the patient should be warned accordingly.

The surgical procedure should follow conventional lines with the raising of buccal and lingual muco-periosteal flaps and the protection of the lingual nerve with the appropriate retractor. Bone should be removed to allow access to the crown and root. If there is any suggestion of danger to the inferior dental nerve, consideration should be given to sectioning the tooth with separate elevation of the crown and roots. Careful debridement and soft tissue closure should then follow.

Retained lower premolar

Like the retained lower wisdom tooth, the retained lower premolar is a common problem. It too can present as a soft-tissue infection (**476**) which, because of its close relationship to the mental nerve may on rare occasions present with altered sensation in the lower lip. It is also a problem to the denture wearer and this again is the usual reason for treatment. As previously mentioned, this tooth lies close to the mental nerve and this is a particular problem during surgery. Careful radiographic examination should indicate the position of the mental foramen in relation to the unerupted tooth

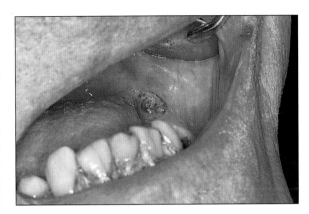

474 Partly erupted retained lower wisdom tooth.

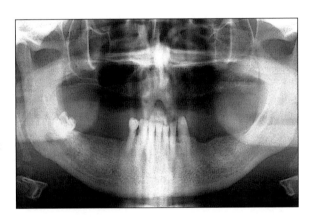

475 Orthopantomograph showing retained lower right wisdom tooth. This tooth is carious, associated with periapical infection and the root is closely related to the inferior dental canal.

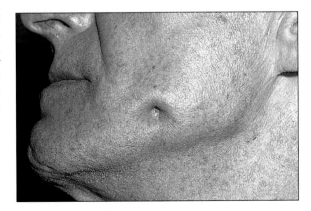

476 Chronic facial sinus arising from an infected retained lower pre-molar.

(**477**). A buccal flap is raised and it is important to identify the mental nerve to allow for its protection during the subsequent procedure. Bone should be carefully removed to expose the tooth, and division of the crown and roots may be required to avoid damage to the nerve. Some postoperative mental paraesthesia may be anticipated as a result of manipulation of the nerve and although recovery may be slow, it should occur within a few weeks or months.

Once again the surgical procedure should be followed by careful debridement and accurate soft-tissue closure. It is often a useful idea to insert the patient's denture postoperatively. This helps to apply some pressure to the surgical area and minimises the postoperative oedema.

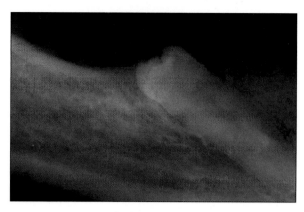

477 Intra-oral radiograph showing the close relationship between a retained lower second pre-molar and the inferior dental canal and mental foramen.

The unerupted maxillary canine

If asymptomatic, these teeth may be left *in situ* and **478** shows a completely unerupted upper left canine which was a chance X-ray finding in a 70-year-old lady. No treatment was thought necessary for this tooth. Sometimes they present a problem to the denture wearer and, in this case, may have to be removed.

Access to the tooth is gained via a buccal flap, or where necessary a palatal flap. Bone removal permits access to the crown and root and the tooth may be simply elevated or removed with upper dental forceps. Debridement and closure are usually followed by the insertion of the upper denture, which can be worn during the immediate postoperative period.

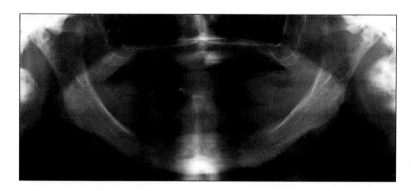

478 Orthopantomograph showing retained unerupted upper left canine.

Facial injuries

The last 20 years have seen changes in the nature of facial injuries. Seat belt and drink/driving legislation has reduced the incidence of major facial injuries as a result of road traffic accidents. Personal assaults now form the commonest cause of jaw fracture. This pattern of injury is mirrored in the elderly population with the added problem of the elderly person's susceptibility to falls. These falls can occur inside or outside the home and may be simple accidents or the result of some underlying medical problem (see Chapter 3). They are a significant cause of facial trauma in the elderly.

Osteoporosis leads to decreased bone density and increased liability to fracture. Consequently, bone behaves more like a dry stick than a green stick and the jaws are no exception. Facial fractures in the elderly are often unstable and reduced muscle tone aggravates this problem. Increased blood vessel fragility means that these fractures may be associated with large haematomas, and gravity allows a gradual spread of bruising along the tissue planes (**479**).

With age, the arterial blood supply to the jaws is reduced and there is also a reduction in the number

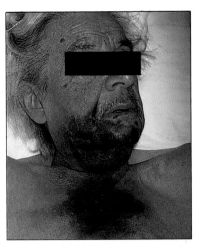

479 Extensive facial bruising as the result of a fractured mandible.

of connective tissue cells within the bone. Consequently, healing of fractures is slow and delayed union and even non-union is a very real problem.

The clinical approach to the elderly trauma patient is based on history and examination. It is important to identify the cause of injury and if a fall is suspected, the nature of the fall needs to be clarified. The cause may have been a simple accident, but possible drug therapy and alcohol problems need to be considered. Medical conditions producing impaired cerebral blood supply, e.g. transient ischaemic attacks, postural hypotension or disturbance of cardiac rhythm, may be involved and further investigation will be needed. Information may be available from relatives or neighbours who will also be able to give an idea of the patient's social circumstances.

Clinical examination should include not only the facial area but extend to exclude fractures elsewhere, e.g. wrist or hip. Radiographs should be taken where appropriate – occipito-mental and lateral views giving a good view of the middle one-third of the face, while panoral and postero-anterior views should be taken for the lower one-third. If there is any suggestion of a blow to the cranium, skull radiographs must be taken and cervical spine views should also be considered.

Decisions regarding management are a balance between potential difficulties for the patient if no treatment is undertaken against the problems involved with admission to hospital, general anaesthesia and the operation itself. Some of the commoner fractures are now considered in more detail.

Mandibular fractures

Condylar fractures are common and by themselves usually need no treatment other than analgesia and encouragement for an early return to function. Angle and body fractures present more of a problem. It may be argued that minimally displaced fractures can be accepted and subsequent adjustments to dentures made to allow for the new position (**480**). However, if there is any significant degree of displacement some form of reduction and fixation will be required. Failure to do so can lead to non-union and permanent disability. Worse still, the unstable fractured segments may ulcerate through the thin oral mucosa and present as an infected compound fracture.

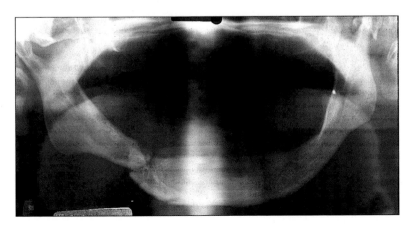

480 Orthopantomograph of a minimally displaced fracture of the right body of the mandible.

Previously, Gunning Splints were constructed from the patients' dentures and the upper and lower splints were used to immobilise the jaws. Widespread use of bone plates has largely superseded this type of fixation. Bone plates can be inserted via intra-oral or extra-oral incisions and this technique allows direct visualisation of the fracture. More precise apposition of the fractured segments can be achieved and there is usually no need for a period of inter-maxillary fixation. Consequently, there is a more rapid return to normal function and this is of particular benefit to the elderly. Bone plates do have a disadvantage in that a degree of periosteal elevation is required to allow their insertion. The periosteum has an important role in the healing of fractures and, in the elderly, it is particularly important to keep this periosteal elevation to a minimum. Prophylactic systemic antibiotics should be used to cover this procedure.

With this technique time in hospital can be reduced, although the patient will need regular postoperative out-patient review. At a later date, superficial bone plates may occasionally ulcerate through the oral mucosa or present a problem beneath the denture flange. If this is the case, it is a simple matter to remove them under local anaesthesia. Some of the above points are illustrated in **481**, **482**. An otherwise fit 70-year-old man who was a driver involved in a road traffic accident is shown in **481**. Clinical and radiographic examination showed a comminuted fracture of the right body of the mandible and a fracture of the left condylar neck. In addition, he sustained a fractured clavicle that required no active treatment. The body fracture of the mandible was plated via an intra-oral incision and good reduction obtained (**482**).

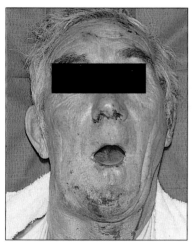

481 Elderly driver involved in road traffic accident, sustaining fractures of the jaw and clavical.

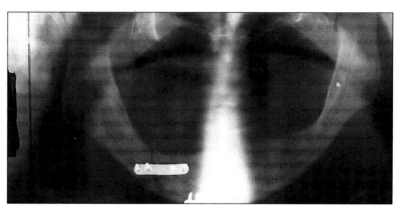

482 Orthopantomograph showing postoperative position following plating of the right body fracture.

Fractures of the zygomatic complex

Patients with fractures of the zygomatic complex may present with periorbital swelling and bruising, flattening of the cheek, subconjunctival haemorrhage and sometimes limitation of mandibular opening. Diplopia may be a problem and the patient may describe infra-orbital paraesthesia.

If soft-tissue swelling allows, clinical examination should include tests of visual acuity and ocular movement. Assessment of the degree of displacement of the zygoma can be made by observation and gentle palpation. A check should also be made on mandibular movement. Occipito-mental radiographs will help confirm the presence of a fracture and also give an indication of the degree of displacement.

Decisions concerning treatment can be delayed for up to 7–10 days, and this allows reduction in soft tissue swelling and easier ophthalmic examination. Diplopia that may have been present often improves as intra-orbital oedema resolves.

Indications for treatment in the elderly are based, in the main, on the restoration of function, with aesthetics of secondary importance. Persistent diplopia and reduced mandibular function would be indications for active management. Less important, but worthy of note, is the problem of infra-orbital paraesthesia; restoration of nerve function is more likely if the fracture has been satisfactorily reduced and an added benefit is that the occasional post-traumatic neuralgia is less likely to be a long-term problem.

General anaesthesia is required for fracture reduction, which is usually carried out via the conventional Gillies approach through a temporal incision. An elevator is used to lift the malar into its original position, but in the elderly this reduction can be unstable and some form of additional fixation may be required. This is commonly achieved by approaching the zygomatico-frontal suture through a lateral eyebrow incision. The insertion of a small bone plate or an interosseous wire across the fracture line should be sufficient to stabilise the whole of the zygoma. This procedure does not take long and the patient is unlikely to be in hospital for more than 2 days. Decisions concerning active management should be aimed at restoring function and will have to be balanced against the patient's general health and quality of life.

A depressed fracture of the malar in a fit 67-year-old man is shown in **483**. Treatment was considered appropriate on the grounds of persistent diplopia and pain, although there was also a marked flattening of the cheek. The reduced fracture was stabilised with a bone plate (**484**).

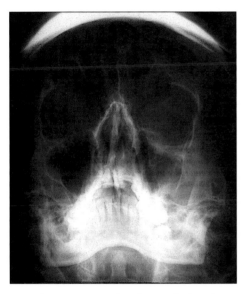

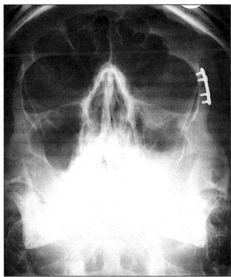

483 Occipito-mental radiograph showing a fracture of the left zygoma.

484 Occipito-mental radiograph showing post-reduction position. The zygoma has been stabilised by a plate at the left zygomatic-frontal suture.

Fractures of the middle one-third of the facial skeleton

Maxillary fractures have become less frequent in the general population and are uncommon in the elderly. They are usually the result of a more serious degree of trauma associated with road traffic accidents or assaults. The patient is likely to present with extensive facial swelling and bruising and the presence of bilateral circum–orbital bruising should always alert the clinician to the possibility of a maxillary fracture (**485**). There may be associated nasal and malar injuries. Gentle manipulation of the maxilla will confirm mobility and give an idea of the degree of displacement. Skull, occipito-mental, lateral facial and panoral radiographs are required to help complete the examination.

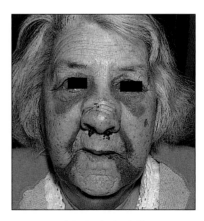

485 An elderly lady following an assault in which she sustained mid-face and nasal fractures.

It is usually possible to avoid active treatment of maxillary fractures in the elderly. Adjustments to full dentures some weeks after the injury can compensate for maxillary displacement as a result of a fracture. More significant to the patient is the implication that an injury of this severity has for their confidence and degree of independence.

Pre-prosthetic Surgery

Pre-prosthetic surgery has gradually expanded its boundaries. It now embraces several more procedures, including the use of skin grafts, osteotomy techniques and the use of bone and hydroxyapatite grafts to restore ridge height, shape and depth. Osseointegrated implants, now widely accepted, will make a significant contribution to this field and are covered in Chapter 12.

For the elderly the aim must be to provide denture comfort with the minimum of surgical interference. It is usually possible to complete these simple procedures under local anaesthesia. The more major procedures outlined above involve general anaesthesia and are probably best reserved for a younger age group. Some of the commonly encountered prosthetic problems will now be considered.

Denture induced hyperplasia

Ill-fitting mobile dentures may produce a hyperplastic reaction within vestibular mucosa and this can occur in either jaw. Acute or chronic ulceration may be superimposed and, very occasionally, the ulcerated lesion may resemble a squamous cell carcinoma. The areas involved vary from small isolated lesions (**486**) to extensive folds of mucosa extending around the entire periphery of the denture (**487**). Primary management should involve considerable reduction in the flange of the denture and this alone can produce a substantial reduction in the size of the lesion, thus minimising the surgery required. Small areas of denture hyperplasia can then be exercised under local anaesthetic. The base of the lesion should be dissected from the underlying tissues using either scalpel, scissors or cutting diathermy. Primary closure is possible, but good results can be obtained by applying a dressing to the denture flange and allowing the surgical wound to granulate. Healing by granulation is associated with scar contraction and, while this is not a problem for smaller lesions, it is a significant difficulty when dealing with extensive hyperplastic areas. The usual procedure in these cases is to excise the hyperplastic tissue and deepen the sulcus at the same time. The raw area is then grafted either with split skin, or less commonly, with mucosa from the oral cavity. Clearly, this is a more extensive procedure and will involve admission to hospital, general anaesthesia and, in the case of skin grafts from the thigh, some temporary reduction in postoperative mobility. Consequently, careful patient selection is required.

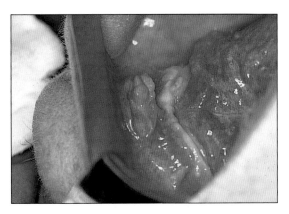

486 Small area of denture induced hyperplasia in the buccal sulcus.

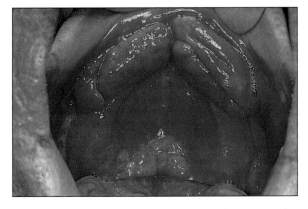

487 Large area of denture hyperplasia obliterating the maxillary buccal sulcus.

Another form of denture-induced hyperplasia is the leaf fibroma (**488**). These are normally found beneath the upper denture and may occasionally reach a large size (**489**). The lesions are pedunculated so that, even in large cases, removal with scalpel or cutting diathermy is simple.

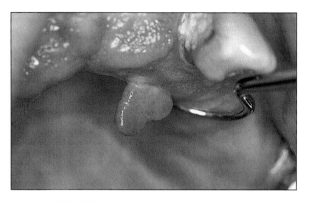

488 Small leaf fibroma.

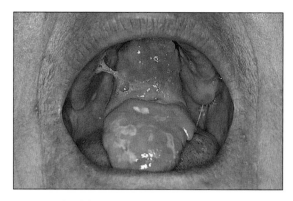

489 Large leaf fibroma. This lesion arises from the incisive papilla and has been displaced downwards onto the tongue for the purposes of the photograph.

The narrow irregular alveolar ridge

This problem is more common in the lower jaw, with the patient experiencing pain as the denture compresses the mucosa against the underlying irregular bone (**490**). This situation is aggravated by denture mobility. If careful attention to the dentures fails to alleviate the problem it is possible to try and improve the situation surgically. This can be done under local anaesthesia and is a relatively simple procedure. An incision is made just on the buccal aspect of the alveolar crest and minimal buccal and lingual flaps are raised to expose the underlying alveolus. Smoothing of the bone can then be performed with bone burs, keeping tissue removal to the minimum consistent with achieving the desired result. This procedure is usually followed by uncomplicated postoperative recovery and the patient can be returned to the prosthodontist.

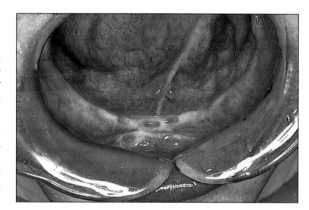

490 Narrow, irregular lower alveolar ridge.

Unsupported alveolar soft tissue

Mobile alveolar soft tissue is usually found in the anterior part of the maxilla and is often the result of wearing a full upper denture opposed by only the lower anterior teeth. This leads to resorption of alveolar bone in the maxilla (**491**) and eventually the anterior nasal spine may become prominent. The clinical result is instability of the upper denture and pain when the nasal spine is traumatised. A variety of

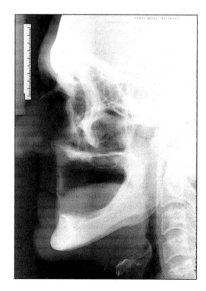

491 Orthopantomograph radiograph showing extensive bone resorption of the maxillary alveolar ridge.

surgical solutions are available for this problem, including ridge augmentation procedures with hydroxyapatite with or without associated vestibuloplasty and skin grafting. This is a major undertaking for the elderly patient and it may be best to consider simple excision of the mobile soft tissue only. This can be done under local anaesthesia – a wedge of tissue is removed from the alveolar crest and the wound edges are undermined and advanced to give the primary closure. This results in considerable reduction of soft tissue mobility. If the anterior nasal spine is a problem this can be reduced at the same operation. These simple procedures involve the minimum upset to the patient and may improve denture stability.

The superficial mental nerve

Resorption of the mandibular alveolus allows the mental foramen to lie close to the alveolar crest (**492**). In some patients, it becomes so superficial that the nerve is traumatised by the denture. This may result in pain, particularly on chewing, or paraesthesia in the distribution of the nerve. This is troublesome to the patient and it is perhaps surprising that it is not more common. If simple easing of the denture fails to resolve the problem, it may be necessary to lower the mental nerve trunk to avoid the trauma from the denture. In order to expose the nerve a mucoperiosteal flap is raised, taking care to keep the crestal incision well to the lingual side. The nerve can then be identified, mobilised and protected. A gutter of bone is removed from below the mental foramen to allow inferior repositioning of the nerve trunk. This procedure requires care and will be followed by a degree of postoperative anaesthesia or paraesthesia. Provided the nerve has not suffered any major trauma, function should eventually return.

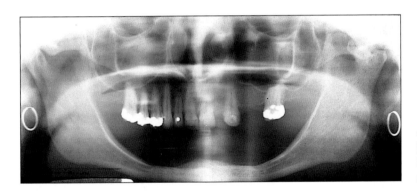

492 Orthopantomograph showing bilateral superficial mental foraminae. Pain was only present on the right side.

Common salivary gland problems

The elderly may suffer from salivary gland disease, the commonest problem being obstruction secondary to calculus formation. The symptoms produced are those of intermittent pain and swelling of the affected gland, usually associated with meals. The submandibular gland is the most commonly involved, although parotid calculi are not unusual.

In the case of the submandibular gland, the stones usually become impacted in the distal part of the duct. They are often palpable in the floor of the mouth and their presence can be confirmed by a lower occlusal radiograph (**493**). Removal of these stones can be achieved by simple dissection under local anaesthesia (**494**). Occasionally, large stones form. **495** shows bilateral calculi in the submandibular ducts of a 78-year-old lady. These were removed under general anaesthesia through intra-oral incisions.

Salivary gland tumours may also present in the elderly, the commonest of these being the pleo-

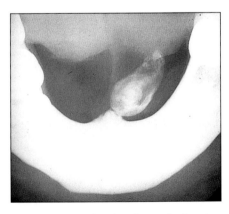

493 Lower occlusal radiograph showing stone impacted in the left submandibular duct.

morphic adenoma. These may arise in the major glands (**496**) or the minor glands (**497**). They are slow growing, usually asymptomatic tumours that may often have been present for many years. More rarely malignant tumours may arise in the major glands. These will usually have a shorter history with associated symptoms, e.g. facial nerve paralysis in malignant parotid tumours.

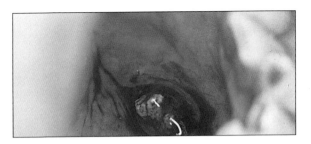

494 Removal of stone from left submandibular duct.

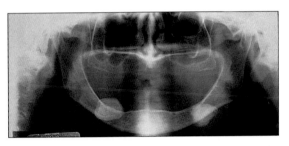

495 Orthopantomograph showing large bilateral submandibular stones.

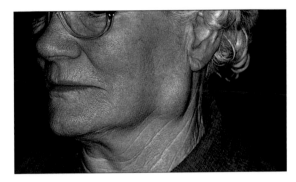

496 Pleomorphic adenoma arising in the left parotid gland.

Malignant Disease

Intra-oral malignancy forms approximately 1% of all reported malignant disease and squamous cell carcinoma represents by far the largest proportion of all oral malignancy. It is more common in older age, with smoking, oral sepsis and alcohol being considered particular risk factors. Early diagnosis is the key to successful treatment and **498** shows a small tumour in the anterior floor of the mouth. This was managed by local resection with every prospect of a cure.

The more advanced the tumour the poorer the prognosis. An ill 70-year-old man presenting with dysphagia and intra-oral pain is shown in **499**. His tongue deviated to the right on protrusion because of the fixation produced by a large tumour. Clinical examination confirmed the presence of a tumour involving the floor of the mouth and the tongue (**500**). Enlarged submandibular lymph nodes were also present. Sadly, with this late presentation the prospects of a cure were poor.

Treatment planning is difficult and decisions are influenced by the site, size and spread of the tumour, the patient's general health and their age. Clearly, full discussion with the patient and their relatives is required.

Surgical excision of the tumour with neck dissection, when appropriate, forms the mainstay of treatment. Modern reconstructive techniques,

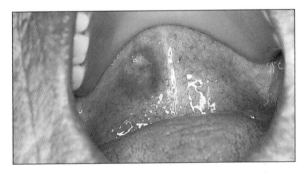

497 Pleomorphic adenoma arising at the junction of the right hard and soft palate.

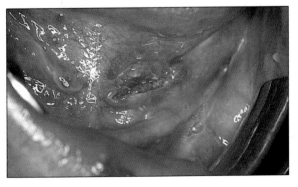

498 Early squamous cell carcinoma, anterior floor of mouth.

particularly the use of 'free flaps', have helped to minimise postoperative morbidity. Radiotherapy may be used to supplement surgery. Decisions to embark on surgical treatment are not undertaken lightly, but it offers the chance of a cure or at least palliation, with improved quality of life in the final stages of the disease.

Finally, when considering oral malignant disease in the elderly it is important to remember the possibility of the mouth being a secondary site for malignant disease elsewhere in the body (**501**). The lungs and breast in particular should be considered as possible primary sites.

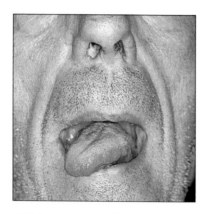

499 Seventy-year-old man with deviation of the tongue on protrusion caused by the large floor of the mouth tumour.

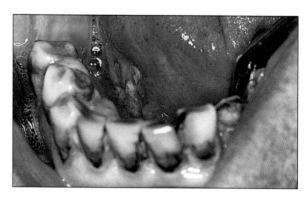

500 Extensive squamous cell carcinoma involving right floor of mouth and tongue.

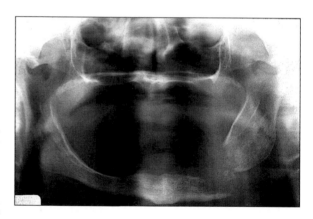

501 Orthopantomograph showing pathological fracture of the left body of the mandible.

Summary

There will be increasing requirement to provide oral surgery services for the elderly and the importance of an understanding approach to the patient and their relatives cannot be underestimated. Careful history taking, including detailed attention to medical problems and concurrent medication, is required. Selection of the appropriate form of anaesthesia is always difficult and an anaesthetist's opinion should be sought if there is any doubt. Finally, and most importantly, treatment plans should be sympathetically tailored to suit the special needs of each individual patient.

Further reading

Davenport, H. 1988. *Anaesthesia and the Aged Patient*. Blackwell Scientific Publications, Oxford.

Ferguson, D.B. 1987. *The Aging Mouth*. Karger, Basel.

Meecham, J.G. & Rawlins, M.D. 1987. A comparison of two different dental local anaesthetic solutions on plasma potassium concentrations. *Anaesthesia*, 191–3.

Shapiro, S., Bomberg, T.J., Benson, B.W. & Harnby C.I. 1985. Post-menopausal osteoporosis: dental patients at risk. *Gerodontics*, **1**, 220–5.

15. Domiciliary Visiting

Domiciliary visiting

The majority of elderly infirm people live within private homes or community residential accommodation. The numbers of such persons who are unable to achieve movement alone increases with age (**502** – adapted from General Household Survey 1986, HMSO 1989).

The home visit to an old person by a health professional is most commonly part of the overall objective in maintaining their independence for as long as possible. The purpose is to arrive at a personal assessment of need and then to present, in a coordinated way, the most suitable help without the creation of additional dependency. It is within the patient's living environment that their total situation, i.e. health, social, economic, is more fully revealed. Caring for elderly disabled persons is a team matter and the dentist is often a neglected member of the multi-disciplinary services that should be made available. The dentist making a home visit will be able to gain therefore, a balanced insight into the conditions that may influence the oral health of the elderly infirm patient. However, oral health care other than pain relief, can be sometimes regarded as of only marginal significance in the aged infirm patient, and even a potential additional burden. This highlights the need for carers to know what dentistry can offer and also for them to act as informed reporters, so that appropriate contact with a dental service can be made. A simple rule is for them to recognise change in habits such as eating, speaking and wearing dental appliances, any of which may be a reflection of oral changes requiring advice. Whoever makes the request for a dental visit, if possible the patient should be informed why it is considered appropriate. An explanatory letter addressed to the patient, detailing the nature and value of the proposed visit, is helpful. In circumstances where a carer may need to read, interpret and act on the communication, a separate covering note to them should be included. The family medical practitioner should always be kept informed of the home service being provided for a particular patient and its objectives (**503**). It is also necessary to have available the up-to-date medical history and any associated therapies.

UNABLE TO ACHIEVE ALONE (%)	65-69	70-74	75-79	80-84	85+
Go Out	5	7	14	24	47
Use Stairs	4	5	10	17	31
Move Around One Level	1	1	2	3	6
Toilet	1	1	2	2	7
In/Out of bed	1	1	3	2	7

502 Some data on disabilities of older people.

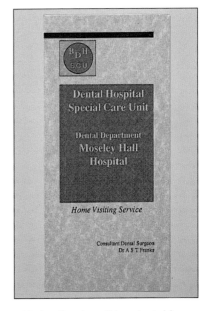

503 Leaflet describing dental home visiting service.

Reasons for domiciliary visiting

While treatment in a dental practice or clinic of a hospital, may be technically desirable, there are a number of possible disadvantages:
- Physical assistance required for moving the disabled person and the special transport.
- Risk during journey to distant clinic through exhaustion, emotional disturbance or infection.
- Elderly disabled patients do not normally suit the tempo of the usual form of dental practice and special sessions devoted to their care may have to be considered.

Patients who benefit from domiciliary care

Home visits are necessary when:
- The patient is too ill or disabled to visit the surgery (including severe visual and hearing loss and problems of incontinence).
- There are carer support problems.
- An assessment visit is requested by a medical colleague, nurse or other professional carer.
- An infirm patient has recently been bereaved.
- Home conditions may influence possible treatment options.

Chronic illness, in addition to physical aspects of disability, also has other repercussions. Often a lack of will develops in the patient and they will not respond to an invitation to visit the surgery or clinic.

Objectives of dental domiciliary visit

The objectives of a dental domiciliary visit are:
- To provide assessment, guidance and treatment to elderly infirm patients.
- To provide information and health education to the client group.
- To support the professional and non-professional carers and participate in the team approach to the concept of total health care.
- To provide sensitive and effective palliative care for the dying patient.

Advantages of domiciliary visiting

The advantages of domiciliary visiting are that:
- The patient is more rested at home with reduced liability towards disorientation. For the frightened patient the home visit can act as a reassuring bridge between home and clinic.
- It allows assessment of home conditions with the level of carer support available. Relatives caring for infirm elderly person often suffer from chronic fatigue and depression. The evidence of an additional area of professional help can contribute much to the maintenance of their own support for their dependent.
- It provides an easier way to check level of medication and prescription compliance; many patients take non-prescription drugs.
- It allows appropriate assessment of self-care levels and of manipulative skills related to oral health.
- The patient may be more confident in accepting advice if they have the territorial advantage.

Disadvantages

The constraints around domiciliary visiting relate mainly to the safety of certain clinical procedures. In addition to standard clinical safeguards, there are some factors that reduce the level of efficiency found in a dental clinic, i.e. lighting, suction, modification of usual working angles. Difficulties with appropriate radiographic facilities can limit diagnosis and certain forms of treatment (e.g. endodontic therapy).

The visit

Following notification of a proposed visit, a telephone call just beforehand is helpful as a reminder to confirm details. Elderly infirm patients require extra time to prepare themselves com-fortably and without anxiety to receive visitors. Appointments are best made avoiding early morning and, as they also fatigue easily, the late evening.

History and diagnosis

An informal atmosphere should be created by the clinician and maintained during the visit (**504**). Where relatives are directly involved in care they can be present during the visit but any discussion should, if possible, take place through the patient (**505**). If consultation with family members or carer alone is indicated, it should be arranged discretely and the patient should not be exposed to needless fear and anxiety. Information from the carers can include any change of habit of oral function or appliance wear and also the state of the appetite, which can often give clues to the ability to use the mouth. On the initial visit, keeping equipment to a minimum will help towards the informal atmosphere. Most elderly infirm patients also gain reassurance from periodic hand contact with the clinician (**506**).

The simple requirements for an initial examination, can include the following: mouth torch and disposable items such as tongue spatulas, gauze, face mask, gloves, alcohol wipe, all of which can be contained in a small plastic bag (**507**).

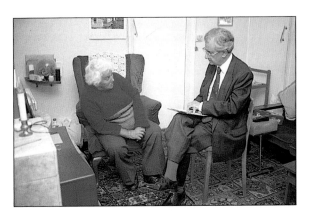

504 An informed and relaxed consultation.

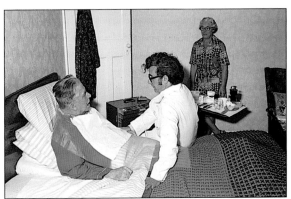

505 If possible, direct discussion with the patient is preferable.

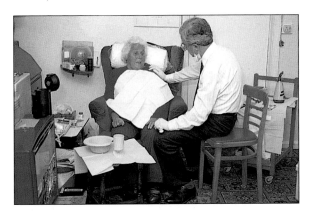

506 Periodic hand contact can be reassuring.

Assessment

At an early point in the first home visit, an explanation should be given to the patient and carers that its purpose is initially to assess the patient's needs. Unrealistic expectations for certain types of dental

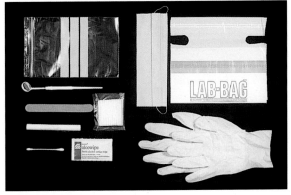

507 Equipment for an initial examination.

treatment and its immediate provision, by members of the family on behalf of the patient, are often the result of lack of communication.

The patient's general functional ability should be evaluated with regard, in particular, to the ability to carry out oral health procedures and to manage the use of any dental appliance. As part of the assessment, the home situation will need to be considered, including care provision, nursing needs and the living environment. Where possible, the patient should be involved in any resultant decision-making and the carers allowed to contribute to discussion of the treatment plan. It is essential to obtain the patient's consent for the dental treatment to be carried out.

Equipment for domicillary visiting

Patient comfort

Arthritic changes affecting the neck and back are very common in the elderly infirm patient and appropriate support is essential during any dental procedures. Neck support cushions can be used for high-backed armchairs (**508**). Domestic seating can be adapted using a portable headrest and backrest (**509**). A specially designed headrest is available for wheelchairs (**510–512**). If a patient is confined to bed, a portable headrest can be fixed to the headboard or to a folding bedrest (**513**).

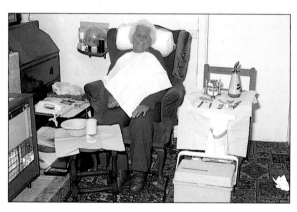

508 Support cushion to achieve a comfortable position for the patient.

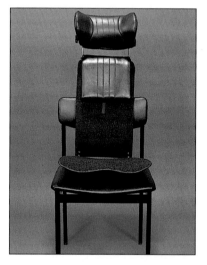

509 A portable head-and back-rest.

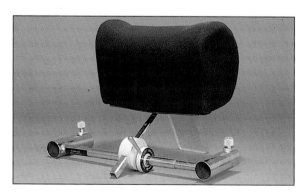

510 A headrest for attachment to a wheelchair.

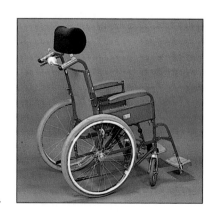

511 Wheelchair with headrest.

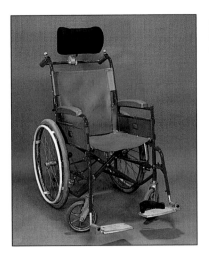

512 With headrest, the wheelchair becomes a good option for dental examination.

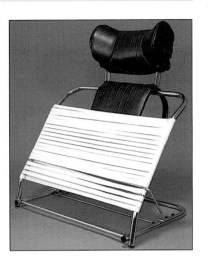

513 A portable back and headrest for a patient restricted to bed.

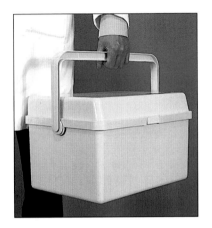

514 A convenient plastic carrying box (designed for a younger age-group!).

Domiciliary kit containers

Lightweight plastic boxes are available which are easy to keep clean, have adequate storage and are inexpensive (**514**, **515**).

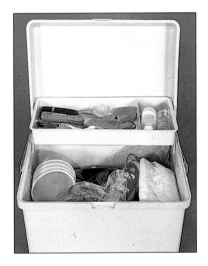

515 Convenient storage.

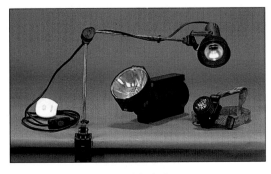

516 A selection of portable lights.

Lighting

Diffuse oral cavity lighting can be provided by a clip-on mains light or large battery torch. A headlight with lens is also useful in order to keep the hands free (**516**), although some patients find the effect off-putting. Intra-oral mirror lights are available with either a battery in the middle or rechargeable components (**517**, **518**).

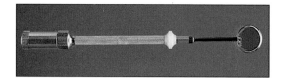

517 A self-contained illuminated mirror.

Pulp tester

Battery pulp testers are available with unitary control by the operator (**519**).

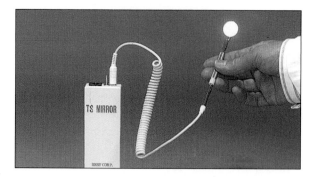

518 Mouth mirror with separate battery-pack.

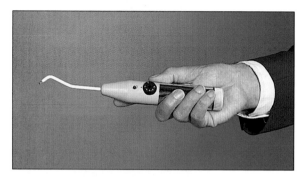

519 Battery operated pulp tester.

Portable engines and aspirators

All electrical equipment with a mains connection used on domiciliary visits should be circuited for safety, through a power breaker. Comprehensive and compact lightweight mobile equipment is now available in fitted cases with separate compressor units (**520–522**). Small lightweight motor units are available for simple procedures. Illustrated are a small hobby motor adequate for denture adjustments (**523**) and a high-speed unit for intra-oral work (**524**). A rechargeable battery/mains operated micromotor is extremely effective for simple tooth-corrective procedures. It has a variable speed control up to 20 000 r.p.m., and the handpieces are autoclaveable (**525, 526**).

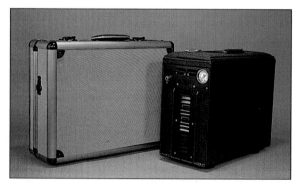

520 Equipment to extend treatment capability.

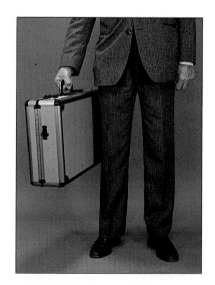

521 A genuinely portable unit.

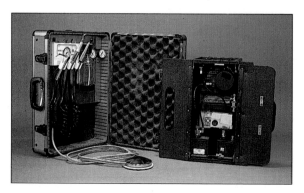

522. Portable units provide much of the surgery capability.

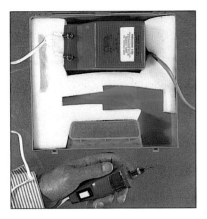

523 A simple electric motor for prosthetics.

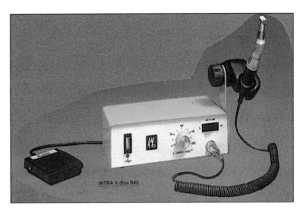

524 A more sophisticated motor for use intra-orally.

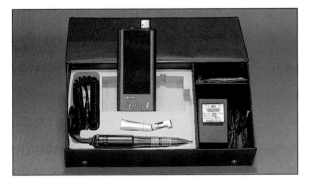

525 Use of rechargeable power source increases convenience of use.

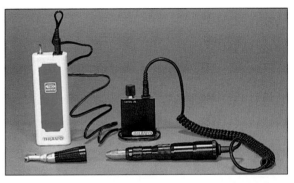

526 High speed and autoclavable handpieces can be employed (see also **525**).

Aspirators and compressed air

Portable aspiration is also available through separate units (**527**, **528**). Compressed air canisters marketed for use on photographic equipment, can be used for prosthetic procedures. However, the pressure control mechanism does not have the precision of flow suitable for intra-oral use (**529**).

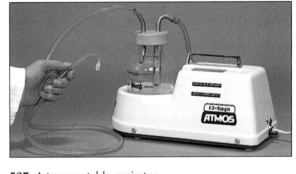

527 A transportable aspirator.

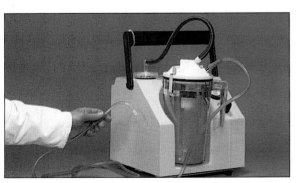

528 Aspiration – an alternative design. Choice will depend upon portability as well as function.

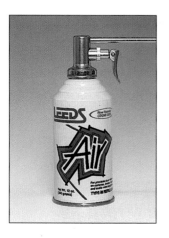

529 A possible source of compressed air.

Wax heaters

Naked flames can ignite easily the latex disposable gloves worn by clinicians. Hot-air blowers are available which provide an even stream of heated air below the ignition point of latex. They work from mains electricity supply and are suitable for most prosthetic procedures (**530**).

Waste disposal

Soiled items must be collected in self-seal plastic laboratory bags (**531**).

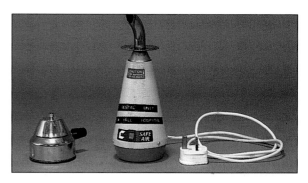

530 An electric hot air device – an alternative to spirit burner (or miniature gas flame).

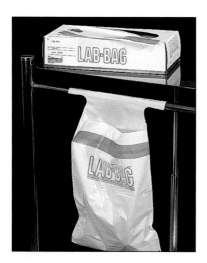

531 Waste collection.

Oral hygiene

The most effective approach to oral hygiene instruction is on an individual basis for which the dental hygienist has appropriate training (**532**). A demonstration of recommended anti-plaque procedures is necessary to supplement the structured guidance (**533**).

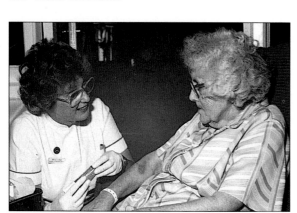

532 A major role for the dental hygienist.

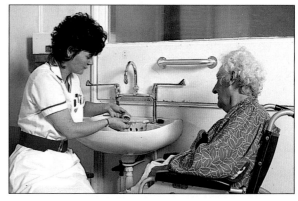

533 Oral hygiene instruction on site.

Many elderly infirm patients have reduced hand function through arthritis (**534**). For such persons, toothbrush handles can be easily and cheaply modified to improve both the ease of use and effectiveness (**535**). Brushes with suction cups for attachment to washbasins can be used one handed (e.g. stroke disabilities) for denture cleaning (**536**).

A range of mouth rinsing-vessels can be tried by the patients (**537**). Tailored help, in addition to improving the effectiveness of and commitment to home care, acts as a powerful encouragement. All patients who require domiciliary visiting also need regular reinforcement of preventive measures from a dental health advisor, perhaps on a 3-month basis.

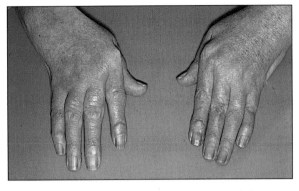

534 Arthritis likely to affect oral hygiene capability.

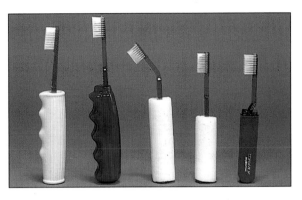

535 Examples of aids to toothbrush manipulation.

536 Denture brushes with suction cups.

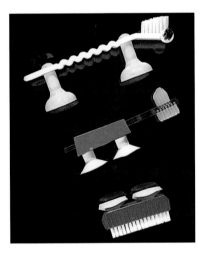

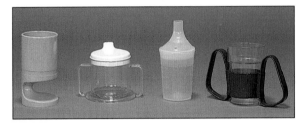

537 Aids to oral rinsing.

Total care patient

The patient who is permanently bedridden may still be able to practise oral hygiene and should be encouraged to do so. If the patient is not able to sit up, the following procedure can be adopted. The patient is placed on their side with the cheek extending over the edge of the pillow. A towel, on which there is a kidney dish, is put under the cheek extending over the side of the bed (**538**). A portable aspirator will also be found to be necessary (**539**).

After brushing the teeth, the inside of the mouth is wiped with a sponge applicator or gauze moistened either in dilute chlorhexidine gluconate (5 ml. of a 1%

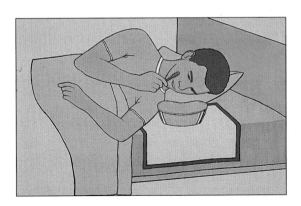

538 Mouth rinsing in bed.

solution in 200 ml water) or sodium bicarbonate solution (1:160) (**540**). The surface of the tongue is also gently cleaned to avoid building up of deposits.

Carers will find a small torch (example fitted with cheek retractor) and plastic mouth mirror helpful (**541**).

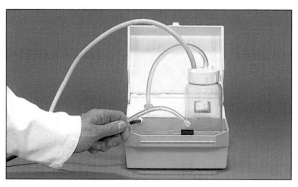

539 Simple suction device.

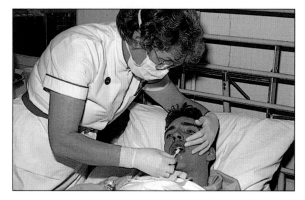

540 Assistance with oral cleansing.

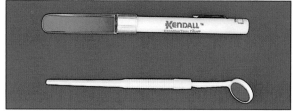

541 Equipment for the carer.

Palliative care

As part of the care of patients who are terminally ill there is a significant place for a dental health input. Oral discomfort may arise as a result of certain forms of chemotherapy, as well as through oral hygiene neglect.

Maintenance of oral health and comfort

Palliative care for a patient may extend over many months. During that time oral health problems may emerge which can cause much additional distress. Many of these additional discomforts can be avoided with care and instruction (**542**). Experience has shown that relatives are often willing to contribute to this aspect of nursing.

Medication

During palliative care, there is often a reduction in salivation. This can contribute to difficulty in swallowing drug tablets. The result is that they can remain against the tissues of the mouth, particularly in the sulcus between the cheek and gum, or underneath the tongue. In these situations an unpleasant ulceration of the mucous membrane can result. Drugs administered in liquid form are

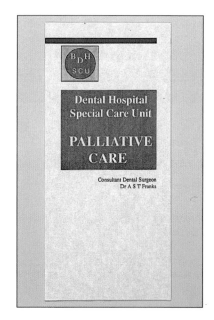

542 Advice on palliative dental care.

preferable, but these are often sweetened and oral hygiene procedures should be emphasized. A refreshing and palatable moisturising aid is an iced lolly made with tonic water. Drying of the oral tissues of a comatose patient is a regular occurrence. Repeated inspection – two or three times a day – is necessary and moisturising agents should be used. Prior to cleaning the mouth, lubrication of the lips is recommended, using a emollient and barrier cream: Dimethicone cream (British National Formulary) or E45 Cream (Crookes Medical Products, U.K.). The following agents can also be usefully employed:

- Mouth cleaners. (a) Sponge applicator, for use with chlorhexidine gluconate, sodium bicarbonate solution or saliva substitute; (b) Moistir® oral swab sticks
- Mouth lubricant. Saliva Orthano® is a saliva substitute that can be used as a spray or on a sponge applicator (**543**).

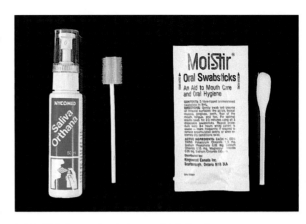

543 Aids for maintaining oral lubrication.

Instruction to carers

The important carers are those who provide day-to-day supervision of the patient and, apart from family, may include neighbours or friends. Carers want and need practical help in looking after the dependent person. Positive contribution by the dentist will promote a cooperative spirit in contributing towards the patient's oral health. Dental hygienists are now able to extend their services to provide a domiciliary service in support of the practitioner. Instructions must be realistic and it has to be emphasised that often the care process for oral health will be continuous and difficult. It is instinctive for relatives and nurses to take over many of the patient's requirements for hygiene, but patients should be allowed to do as many things as possible for themselves in order to reduce dependency. Simple instruction pamphlets should be available for distribution to the families of elderly infirm patients (**544**).

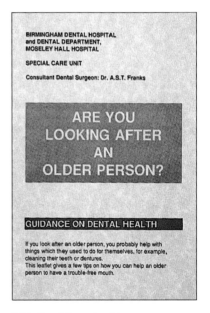

544 Provision of guidance to carers.

Further reading

Christensen, J. 1988. Domiciliary care for the elderly patient. *Dental Update*, **15**, 284.

Ettinger, R.L. 1977. Dental care for the housebound: assessment and hygiene. *Australian Dental Journal,* **22**, 77.

Franks, A.S.T. & Hedegard B. 1973. *Geriatric Dentistry.* Blackwell Scientific Publications, Oxford.

Kesner, A. 1981. Geriatric dentistry in the nursing home. *New York State Dental Journal*, **47**, 199.

Shaver, R.O. 1985. Delivery systems for the housebound dental patient. In *Clinical Geriatric Dentistry*, ed. H.H. Chauncey. American Dental Association, Chicago.

Index

Page numbers in *italics* refer to illustrations and tables